"Mentoring in Healthcare *redefines mentorship as a culture-building strategy, not a checkbox activity. This book is crucial reading for anyone managing scientists, medical affairs, or clinical development teams.*" — **Jon R. Cohen, MD, CEO, Talkspace, Prior CEO and Executive Chairman, BioReference Laboratories, and Prior Chief Medical Officer, Northwell Health System**

"*A welcome addition to the mentorship canon—robust enough for academic discourse, practical enough for real life use.*" — **Christine Laine, MD, MPH, Editor-in-Chief, *Annals of Internal Medicine*, Senior Vice President, American College of Physicians, and Professor of Medicine, Sidney Kimmel Medical College, Thomas Jefferson University**

"Mentoring in Healthcare *brilliantly integrates the inspirational with the practical. The authors have creatively leveraged evidence and their experience to build a toolkit applicable in the real world.*" — **Namita Seth Mohta, MD, Executive Editor, *NEJM Catalyst* and Assistant Professor, Harvard Medical School**

"Mentoring in Healthcare *fills the gap between good intentions and great mentorship. As both a practicing physician and entrepreneur, I've seen countless well-meaning attempts at mentorship fall short due to lack of structure and proven frameworks. Ruth, Vineet, and Sanjay provide the practical tools and evidence-based strategies that transform casual guidance into transformative career development.*" — **Scott Parazynski, MD, Astronaut, Explorer, Serial Entrepreneur, and Author of *The Sky Below***

"*Grounded in real-world experience,* Mentoring in Healthcare *is an indispensable resource for cultivating the next generation of healthcare leaders. It is a compelling guide that demystifies the art and science of mentorship with clarity, wisdom, and heart.*" — **Brian P. Bosworth, MD, FACG, Chief Medical Officer, NYU Langone Health and Professor of Medicine, NYU Grossman School of Medicine**

"*A thoughtful, evidence-informed guide to what effective mentorship looks like in real life. This book fills a long-standing gap in academic medicine with clarity, honesty, and practical wisdom.*" — **Talia H. Swartz, MD, PhD, Senior Associate Dean for MD-PhD Education, Director, Medical Scientist Training Program, Associate Professor of Medicine, Icahn School of Medicine at Mount Sinai, Co-Chair, AAMC Group on Research Education and Training Steering Committee, and Chair, AAMC Group on Research Education and Training, MD-PhD Steering Committee**

"*As someone with experience leading training programs for MD/PhD and PhD trainees as well as medical residents and fellows, I find* Mentoring in Healthcare *an essential resource. It highlights the importance of preparation, clear expectations, and collaborative mentorship, offering practical strategies to foster meaningful and productive mentor-mentee relationships.*" — **Robin G. Lorenz, MD, PhD, Executive Director, Research Pathology, Genentech**

"*Finally—a book on mentoring that won't just collect dust on my shelf! Thoughtful, practical, and refreshingly honest, this is a must-read for anyone serious about patient safety, healthcare quality, or simply not repeating their own early-career mistakes. I'll be recommending it widely (and possibly assigning it).*" — **John M. Hollingsworth, MD, MSc, Chief Quality Officer, UF Health Shands Hospital and UF Health Physicians and Professor of Urology, University of Florida College of Medicine**

"*Empowering, practical, and deeply relevant to real-world mentoring challenges in all healthcare fields. Ruth Gotian, Vineet Chopra, and Sanjay Saint understand the realities of frontline mentorship—and it shows.*" — **Milisa Manojlovich, PhD, RN, Professor of Nursing, University of Michigan School of Nursing and Co-Director for the National Clinician Scholars Program, University of Michigan**

"*Mentorship is the fuel of the most successful career engines. This book gives us a look under the hood and turn-by-turn instructions needed for great mentors, mentees, and mentoring teams.*" — **Kimberly D. Manning, MD, MACP, FAAP, Professor of Medicine, Vice Chair, RYSE Initiatives, Emory University Department of Medicine**

"*This book takes mentoring from something we talk about to something we can truly excel at!*" — **Allen Kachalia, MD, JD, Senior Vice President, Patient Safety and Quality, Director, Armstrong Institute for Patient Safety and Quality, Johns Hopkins Medicine**

"*In my long career, the accomplishment I am most proud of is advice, help, and support I have given to several thousand people who I taught, trained, collaborated with, or mentored. Some of these relationships have lasted for years. As a result, I frequently say, 'You are now a guest at the Detsky Hotel California. You can check out any time you like, but you can never leave.' This book will give mentors and mentees all the practical tools they need to be successful. Keep it on your shelf for a long time.*" — **Allan S. Detsky, MD, PhD, CM, Professor, University of Toronto**

"Mentoring in Healthcare *gives both voice and a practical structure to something every healthcare leader greatly values: helping faculty, staff, and trainees succeed. The valuable lessons from this easy-to-ready book are highly relevant in healthcare settings throughout the world.*" — **Alessandro Bartoloni, MD, Professor of Infectious Diseases, University of Florence and Director of Infectious and Tropical Diseases, Careggi University Hospital, Florence, Italy**

"Mentoring in Healthcare *elevates mentorship as a leadership imperative among healthcare workers throughout the world. I was especially struck by the discussion of sacred moments in mentoring relationships—it is a simple yet powerful message.*" — **Anucha Apisarnthanarak, MD, President, Asia Pacific Society of Infection Control, Professor and Chief of Infectious Diseases Division, Thammasat University Hospital, Bangkok, Thailand**

"Mentoring in Healthcare *is an essential resource for anyone in healthcare committed to fostering growth, excellence, mindfulness, and resilience in themselves and their colleagues. This book offers strategies and wisdom that will empower both mentors and mentees to build meaningful, transformative relationships.*" — **Yasuharu Tokuda, MD, MPH, PhD, Director, Muribushi Okinawa Center for Teaching Hospitals, Okinawa, Japan**

"*Essential reading for those of us responsible for developing the next generation of clinician-scholars and healthcare leaders. This book—written by experts in three leading U.S. medical schools—effectively translates mentoring from art to science.*" — **Akihiko Saitoh, MD, PhD, Professor and Chairman of Pediatrics, Vice Dean, Niigata University School of Medicine, Niigata, Japan**

Mentoring in Healthcare

Mentoring in Healthcare: The Definitive Guide to Cultivating Individual and Organizational Success is a focused guide to help strengthen mentorship relationships and refine the experience for healthcare professionals. It addresses the pressing need for effective mentorship amid current challenges such as burnout, workforce shortages, and funding restrictions.

Targeted at a wide range of healthcare professionals—from trainee to executive—the book emphasizes the vital role of mentorship in professional development and success, illustrating the transformative journey from student to accomplished healthcare professional.

Authored by Ruth Gotian, EdD, MS, Vineet Chopra, MD, MSc, and Sanjay Saint, MD, MPH, MACP, this book draws on their extensive backgrounds in academic medicine. With evidence-based strategies informed by the authors' research and experience, *Mentoring in Healthcare* fills a gap in the existing literature, offering actionable advice to help healthcare professionals succeed.

Mentoring in Healthcare

The Definitive Guide to Cultivating Individual and Organizational Success

Ruth Gotian, EdD, MS

Vineet Chopra, MD, MSc

Sanjay Saint, MD, MPH, MACP

CRC Press
Taylor & Francis Group
Boca Raton London New York

CRC Press is an imprint of the
Taylor & Francis Group, an **informa** business

First edition published 2026
by CRC Press
2385 NW Executive Center Drive, Suite 320, Boca Raton, FL 33431

and by CRC Press
4 Park Square, Milton Park, Abingdon, Oxon, OX14 4RN

CRC Press is an imprint of Taylor & Francis Group, LLC

ISBN: 978-1-041-00710-4 (hbk)
ISBN: 978-1-041-00693-0 (pbk)
ISBN: 978-1-003-61123-3 (ebk)

DOI: 10.1201/9781003611233

Typeset in Bembo
by Apex CoVantage, LLC

For the mentors who guided me, the mentees who inspired me, and my cherished family who supported me. In blessed memory of my parents, Dina and Arthur Ginsburg, z'l, whose legacy lives on every page.

Ruth Gotian

To my many mentors, coaches, sponsors, and connectors, and to the many mentees who have shaped me today—thank you for your endless support and wisdom.

Vineet Chopra

To my parents, Prem and Raksha Saint—the best mentors I could ever wish for.

Sanjay Saint

Contents

Contents

Foreword

Early in my tenure as the Director of the Duke Clinical Research Institute and seeking to better understand how to shape a successful research career, I sent around a simple survey to the institute's faculty. I asked, "What does an early career investigator and a senior investigator need for a successful career?" The results were clear, and it was not surprising to me that mentorship was the top answer to both questions. Mentorship in healthcare, in both research and clinical careers, is critical. As this book's thoughtful authors recognize, so much of clinical care and scientific training is unwritten and experiential. In healthcare's working and learning environments, having colleagues (both peers and those in more senior roles) who devote their energy to providing guidance, support, and insights into a career can be the difference between success and struggle.

During my own professional journey, now across three medical schools as a faculty member (Duke, Stanford, and Weill Cornell), I have mentored dozens of students, trainees, faculty, and staff with a personal style and approach that was heavily influenced by what my many mentors taught me. Three mentors especially influenced my career, including sometimes difficult choices that I made along the way. When I sought certain types of training, to assume new responsibilities, or to consider leadership opportunities that twice involved cross-country moves, they provided valuable guidance. From supporting my professional (and personal) growth over decades, my closest mentors are now both colleagues and friends. Today we are a team with shared values and often goals.

Mentors with different skillsets and diverse areas of expertise, even a spectrum of personality types, can help with exploring problems, challenges, and opportunities that a healthcare career offers. From one mentor, whom I met at age 21, I learned the importance of "paying it forward," and this helped establish my own commitment to mentoring. The second mentor, whom I met when I was a cardiology fellow, taught me the importance of data-driven decision-making and the criticality of not compromising one's value system when making those decisions. The third mentor is an international colleague whom I met as a research fellow in cardiology; in an uncertain world, he continues to impress upon me the importance of grace, respect, dignity, and civility in professional interactions and activities. This mentorship from them and others has given me a framework for how I interact with my own mentees. As the survey said, mentors lead us to career success, to be better if not best.

The authors of *Mentoring in Healthcare*, senior leaders and experienced educators and mentors from three academic health systems and representing the geographic spread of the United States, from the east coast to the west, have distilled their experiences, their observations of others, and the mentoring literature into a clear, succinct, easy-to-use, three-part guide for mentors, mentees, and the mentor–mentee team. They tackle the complexities of these very human relationships and provide paths that we can all take to succeed.

As I continue on my own professional journey in healthcare as both a mentor and a mentee, I am still learning. Take my advice and do not fail the reading test. Read on. Like everything else we learn in medicine, be it taking a history or performing a procedure, mentoring is a skill that can be taught, learned, and refined. Consider mentoring and being mentored as lifelong opportunities with lifelong rewards!

Robert A. Harrington, MD
Stephen and Suzanne Weiss Dean, Weill Cornell Medicine
Provost for Medical Affairs, Cornell University

Preface

No one builds a successful career alone—not in medicine, not in science, and certainly not in healthcare. Yes, rigorous training, unyielding curiosity, and the relentless drive to keep learning are critical components. But behind every confident decision in the clinic, every bold step in research, and every new leadership role is someone who believed in us long before and more than we believed in ourselves. That's mentorship.

Mentorship is not a luxury. It's the hidden engine behind the most impactful healthcare careers. At its core, mentorship is a relationship between someone with experience and insight and someone eager to learn, grow, and lead. It's how we pass down not just the written but also the unwritten curriculum—the norms, values, culture, and nuances they don't teach in school or write about in textbooks. These are the workarounds built on late nights and second chances. And in healthcare, where the stakes are high and the learning never ending, mentorship isn't optional. It's essential.

The best mentorship relationships are reciprocal. Yes, mentees gain confidence, skills, and clarity. But mentors? They gain purpose, perspective, and the chance to shape the future of their field. They also learn new skills and a wealth of lived experience in managing relationships. Mentorship becomes their legacy as the ripple effect of one strong mentoring relationship can live on for generations.

But let's be honest. Mentorship can also go wrong, very wrong. We've seen relationships built on the best of intentions leave a trail of collateral damage. Mismatched expectations have led to resentment or regret. In some egregious cases, what started as support morphed into what we call mentorship malpractice—when a mentor does more harm than good and turns into a tormentor. We feel these stories are equally important to share, because we learn just as much from the failures as we do from the successes, perhaps more.

We've spent much of our careers researching, teaching, writing about, and practicing mentoring. We've mentored students, residents, fellows, faculty, and academic leaders. And we continue to be mentored by others. We've interviewed hundreds of professionals in healthcare and beyond, from Nobel Prize winners to department chairs, deans, C-suite leaders, residents, and nurses, about what makes mentoring in healthcare work.

This book is the blueprint for all mentors and mentees in healthcare. It distills what we've learned, taught, and practiced into actionable, evidence-informed guidance. You'll find practical strategies for building strong mentoring relationships, avoiding common traps, and navigating challenges unique to the healthcare environment. To reach every learner, we've added scripts, worksheets, checklists, and workflows to guide you every step of the way, as well as supplemental resources.

Whether you're an experienced mentor, a brand-new mentee, someone juggling both roles (as many in healthcare do), or a leader in healthcare, this book is for you. We hope it will help you build meaningful, effective, and enduring mentoring relationships. Because when we get mentorship right, we don't just advance careers. We improve lives.

Ruth Gotian, EdD, MS
New York, New York
Vineet Chopra, MD, MSc
Denver, Colorado
Sanjay Saint, MD, MPH, MACP
Ann Arbor, Michigan

Acknowledgments

In 2018, the three of us—Ruth, Vineet, and Sanjay—first crossed paths through a (you guessed it) mentoring program. What began as a serendipitous connection quickly turned into mutual respect and admiration. Over the years, we kept in touch, watching each other's work and scholarship on mentoring evolve and expand. In early 2020, we said, "Let's write a book together." Then the world shut down. The idea was shelved, but not forgotten. Fast forward to 2023: reunited (again through a mentoring program, of course), we knew it was finally time.

Over the next year and half, we immersed ourselves in shaping this book—not just as a collection of ideas, but as something distinct from anything we had written before. We saw a widening hole and variety in the quantity and quality of mentorship within academic medicine and wanted to help close the gap. We understood that what was missing was pragmatic "how to" and "what next" advice. And with the generosity of our mentors, colleagues, and friends, whose insights and encouragement made all the difference, we brought that vision to life.

Ruth is deeply grateful to the mentors who helped her carve her own unique path at every step of her career, especially Drs. Bert Shapiro, Marie Volpe, and Marshall Goldsmith, each of whom encouraged her to lead with curiosity and conviction (and ignore the naysayers). Thank you to the extraordinary colleagues at Weill Cornell Medicine (WCM), some of whom she's had the privilege of working with for nearly three decades. A heartfelt thank you to Drs. Hugh Hemmings and Kane Pryor from WCM's Department of Anesthesiology, for their steadfast support, and to the powerhouse that is the Women's Mentoring Circle for modeling what community in academia should look like.

Special thanks to Eric Schurenberg, a brilliant editor and generous thought partner, who reminded Ruth of the value of focus—and who gently nudged her to zero in on mentoring in healthcare, a much-needed conversation that wasn't being had.

And finally, to Ruth's ultimate support system: Amnon, Benjamin, Jonathan, and Eitan. Thank you for not even blinking when I came home (again) and said, "I'm writing another book." Thank you for the quiet, the space, the endless Nespresso pods, and the tech support always just a text away. To Ron and Daniel, thank you for your patience as your sister tackles yet another project. And to my beloved parents, Dina and Arthur, z'l—how I wish you could have held this book in your hands.

Vineet would like to thank his many clinical and research mentors who saw in him what he did not see in himself at a nascent stage of his career. He is deeply grateful to Dr. Erdal Cavusoglu, Dr. Sanjay Saint, Dr. Larry McMahon, and Dr. Scott Flanders, who played instrumental roles in shaping his thinking about academic medicine. Behind Vineet's success is an incredible family who has loved and supported him no matter the challenge or outcome. They are the most important ingredient of his success.

Sanjay would like to thank Dr. Deb Grady (first research mentor), Dr. Larry Tierney (first clinical mentor), Dr. Bob Wachter (first career mentor), and Drs. Steve Fihn, Ben Lipsky, Larry McMahon, Eve Kerr, Rod Hayward, John Carethers, Gil Omenn, Scott Flanders, Sarah Krein, Tim Hofer, and Jim Woolliscroft. He would also like to acknowledge the University of Michigan and the VA Ann Arbor Healthcare System—two organizations in which mentoring is a core value. Karen Fowler, Latoya Kuhn, Jessica Ameling, Jason Engle, Jinae Stoudemire, Erica Bower, Chris Lozier, John Frye, Martha Quinn, and Michele Mazlin have provided the critical project and administrative support for our research and mentoring programs. Finally, he would like to thank his incredibly supportive and loving family.

Ruth, Vineet, and Sanjay are deeply grateful to their literary agent, Scott Miller of Gray + Miller Agency, for the countless calls, creative strategy sessions, and the honest conversations that pushed this project to the next level. Thank you to Drew Young for his steady patience and unwavering persistence, and to Tony DiCostanzo for ensuring every "i" was dotted and every "t" was crossed with precision. Thank you to Jo Koster at Taylor & Francis for understanding our vision. We also appreciate the personal contributions from Heather Gilmartin, RJ Schildhouse, and Martha Quinn that began several of the chapters. Finally, a huge heartfelt thank you to

Rachel Ehrlinger, who kept us organized, focused, and on schedule: we simply couldn't have done this book without you.

Co-authoring a book is never easy—especially when all three authors hold demanding jobs and live in different cities. But from the beginning, this collaboration was grounded in a shared belief that, together, we could create something stronger, deeper, and more impactful than any one of us could achieve alone. This book is the result of that synergy; it is more than the sum of its parts.

Most of all, we are grateful to one another—for the trust, the friendship, the accountability, and the shared commitment that made this book not only possible but meaningful.

Authors

Dr. Ruth Gotian is Chief Learning Officer and Associate Professor of Education in Anesthesiology at Weill Cornell Medicine, where she served as the inaugural Assistant Dean for Mentoring and as Executive Director of the Mentoring Academy. For over two decades, she directed the Weill Cornell/Rockefeller/Sloan Kettering Tri-Institutional MD-PhD Program, one of the nation's leading physician-scientist training initiatives.

An internationally recognized expert in mentorship, leadership development, and the science of high performance, Dr. Gotian has been named one of the top 20 mentors in the world by the International Federation of Learning and Development, the #1 emerging management thinker by Thinkers50, and one of the Top 50 executive coaches globally. Her work has been featured in the *Wall Street Journal* and on *NBC News*, and she is a LinkedIn Top Voice in Mentoring.

Dr. Gotian has published in leading peer-reviewed journals, including *Academic Medicine, Nature, British Journal of Anaesthesia, JAMA Open*, and the *Journal of Clinical Investigation*. She is also a prolific contributor to *Harvard Business Review, Forbes, Fast Company*, and *Psychology Today*, where she shares evidence-based strategies for optimizing success and cultivating leadership.

She serves on the Board of the American Physician–Scientist Association, was appointed to the Advisory Committee to the Deputy Director for Intramural Research at the National Institutes of Health, is on the Harvard Business Review Advisory Council, and is Associate Editor for the *British Journal of Anaesthesia*.

Dr. Gotian is the award-winning author of *The Success Factor*, and the co-author of the *Financial Times Guide to Mentoring* and a textbook on medical education. Her research focuses on the habits and mindset of elite performers—including Nobel Prize winners, astronauts, Olympians, and NBA champions—and has influenced professionals and organizations around the world. Her scholarship even inspired a theme song: "I'm Possible."

You can learn more about Dr. Ruth Gotian at ruthgotian.com.

Dr. Vineet Chopra is Professor of Medicine, holder of the Robert W. Schrier Endowed Chair, Chairman of the Department of Medicine, and Executive Vice Dean (Interim), all at the University of Colorado (CU). Prior to coming to CU in 2021, Chopra served as the inaugural Chief of the Division of Hospital Medicine at the University of Michigan from 2017 to 2021. A career hospitalist, Chopra's research and clinical interests are dedicated to improving the safety of hospitalized patients by preventing hospital-acquired conditions. He has published almost 300 peer-reviewed publications in top journals, including the *Annals of Internal Medicine, JAMA, NEJM, BMJ*, and others. He has also edited and authored five textbooks, including the *Saint–Chopra Guide to Internal Medicine, The Mentoring Guide, Thirty Rules for Healthcare Leaders*, and *Preventing Hospital Infections*, many of which have been translated into other languages. He presently serves as Deputy Editor at the *Annals of Internal Medicine*, one of the premier internal medicine journals in the world.

Chopra is the recipient of numerous teaching, service, and research awards. He was selected as the recipient of the Kaiser Permanente Award for Clinical Teaching Excellence from the UM Medical School, the Jerome W. Conn Award for Outstanding Research, the Richard D. Judge Award for Medical Student Teaching, and the H. Marvin Pollard Award for outstanding teaching of residents. He received the Society of Hospital Medicine Excellence in Research Award and the Blue Cross/Blue Shield McDevitt Award for Research Excellence. In recognition of his mentoring efforts, he was named a Distinguished Clinical and Translational Research Mentor by the University of Michigan Medical School.

Dr. Sanjay Saint is the Chief of Medicine at the VA Ann Arbor Healthcare System, George Dock Professor of Internal Medicine at the University of Michigan, and Executive Director for the Sacred Moments Initiative.

He is an expert in patient safety with a focus on why some hospitals are better than others at preventing hospital-acquired complications. He has authored over 400 peer-reviewed papers, with nearly 120 appearing in the *New England Journal of Medicine, JAMA, Lancet*, or the *Annals of Internal Medicine*. He serves on the editorial board of seven peer-reviewed journals, including *NEJM Catalyst* and *BMJ Quality & Safety*, and is an elected member of the

American Society for Clinical Investigation (ASCI) and the Association of American Physicians (AAP).

He has written for the *Wall Street Journal* and *Harvard Business Review* and has given a TEDx talk on culture change in healthcare. He has co-authored several books published by Oxford University Press, including *Teaching Inpatient Medicine: Connecting, Coaching, and Communicating in the Hospital* (Second Edition) and *The Saint–Chopra Guide to Inpatient Medicine* (Fifth Edition). He has also co-authored three books published by the University of Michigan: *Thirty Rules for Healthcare Leaders*, *The Mentoring Guide: Helping Mentors and Mentees Succeed*, and *Pickleball for Life: Prevent Injury, Play Your Best & Enjoy the Game*. In 2016, he received the Mark Wolcott Award from the Department of Veterans Affairs as the National VA Physician of the Year and was elected as an International Honorary Fellow of the Royal College of Physicians (FRCP). In 2017, he was awarded the National Health System Impact Award from the Department of Veterans Affairs, and the Distinguished Mentor Award from the University of Michigan. He has been named a Master of the American College of Physicians (MACP), and received the 2023 Under Secretary Award from the Department of Veterans Affairs as the National Health Services Researcher of the Year and the 2023 Michigan Medicine Alumni Society's Distinguished Service Award.

He received his Medical Doctorate from UCLA, completed a medical residency and chief residency at the University of California at San Francisco (UCSF), and obtained a Master's in Public Health (as a Robert Wood Johnson Clinical Scholar) from the University of Washington in Seattle. He has been a visiting professor at over 100 hospitals and universities in the United States, Europe, and Asia.

Becoming an Inspiring Mentor

PART

1

Becoming an Inspiring
Mentor

1

Three Steps to Getting Started as a Mentor

I had just started my career development award and was establishing relationships with my mentors when one of my colleagues in our center's postdoctoral fellowship asked me a surprising question: "Would you be my mentor?" After making sure I heard her correctly, my imposter syndrome reared its ugly head. "You're not senior enough," I heard echoing in my brain. "She's smarter than you and works in a totally different field. What do you have to offer?" was the next thought. I was about to thank her for the lovely request and bow out due to busyness when I stopped and took a deep breath. My inner confidence spoke up, and I heard, "Ask her why?"

I did, and learned she hoped to tap into skills and experiences that I took for granted. We set a first meeting where she outlined how I would fit into her mentoring team and set a game plan. We have been working together for over two years, and she recently submitted her own career development award. I am now a seasoned mentor and will always look back at that first request as my favorite because it was when I found my confidence and asked, "Why me?"

—Heather Gilmartin, PhD, NP, University of Colorado

You have knowledge to share, people look to you for guidance, and, by desire or circumstance, you find yourself mentoring others. Whether you have the coveted "mentor" title or not, you are fulfilling the role. And you need to be ready for this new phase of your career. Sooner or later, someone will ask you to help them grow in an area where you have expertise. Whether that involves a pre-med college student, a surgical trainee, a junior attending, or a new department chair, sharing wisdom, experiences, and shortcut and helping carry emotionally charged experiences are all woven into the fabric of mentorship.

While formal definitions of mentorship vary, traditionally, it is thought of as a reciprocal relationship in a work environment between a more senior person (mentor) and a junior person (mentee) that will ideally benefit both people. For some, this responsibility might occur sooner than expected. Younger fields, such as hospital medicine, must develop mentors at an earlier stage of their career. For others, the role of mentor may come later, once a career has been established, and influence and visibility secured with diverse and varied experiences along the way.

Regardless of timing, becoming well-versed in how effective mentorship works will help you become a better mentor and will catapult your mentee's success. In addition to being both fulfilling and rewarding, a successful mentoring relationship can also help people whom you have not even met, as the perspectives, skills, and behaviors of your mentees will then influence their own mentees, leading to a ripple effect of positive mentoring experiences. As you embark on your mentoring journey, we recommend keeping these three basic steps in mind.

Step 1. Build a Mentoring Team

If you've ever been to the operating room, you know that nothing happens until a team of individuals comes together and goes through a checklist.[1] This is done to prevent medical errors. The idea for this checklist was adopted from airline pilots. It's what they use before any takeoff, landing, or unexpected events. A problem in one industry was solved with a solution from another. This is one of the key benefits of expanding your sphere of awareness. This principle holds true for the art of mentorship.

Gone are the days when having one mentor who was generally older, more senior, and in your exact specialty assured career success. In an era of team science, collaborative breakthroughs, and cross-dimensional thinking, a single mentor limits growth and development. In the traditional mentorship dyad, your mentee is exposed to only one path traveled and the network of only one person. Further complicating the issue, a mentor of a different upbringing, religion, or cultural heritage may not understand or be able to empathize with the nuances of your beliefs and journey. After all, a mentee's definition of success will likely evolve and will need to be shaped by more than one expert.

A mentoring team[2] has become the new standard as it can offer far more benefits than a single mentor, even if that mentor is adorned with achievements and accolades. In the past, a single mentor took a mentee "under their wing" and claimed sole responsibility for a mentee's success. But academic medicine and healthcare have changed, demands on people's time have evolved, and, very often, individuals can no longer control their own schedules. In today's competitive era of team-based problem solving and science, having a sole mentor can be risky, especially for the mentee. Furthermore, it limits the access and perspectives the mentee can gain.

Here are some reasons why team-based mentoring is ideal:

- **The mentee gains a broader perspective:** Different backgrounds, personalities, work styles, experiences, networks, and opportunities for learning are more likely to be realized from a group of people. A sole mentor teaches only their way of doing things, based on their experiences, and deprives the mentee of critical exposure to diversity of thought, creativity, and problem-solving ability. Not to mention, different mentors have varying clinical or methodological skills, career experiences, and areas of expertise. Having a team of mentors—all of whom bring unique talents, networks, and abilities—is key to a mentee's success.

  Consider including mentors who are senior to you and come from various disciplines and institutions. Some may be very senior to you and have leadership roles—such as a department head or someone in the C-suite—in your organization while others are just one rung above you (e.g., a newly promoted associate professor). You may also want to consider near peers (i.e., those just a few years ahead of you), provided their success seems highly likely, to avoid undue competition over first-authorship or recognition on grants. As you work with these mentors, it is likely you will also grow in your skills and abilities.

- **Good mentoring takes time. Having a team ensures the primary mentor gets a more manageable workload:** In today's healthcare setting, plagued by shortened time with patients, increased time on electronic health records, and competing demands, time is a limited resource. Few have the necessary reserves to truly invest in a mentee the way they deserve.

  As the saying goes: "If you want something done, ask a busy person to do it." Much like a rubber band, you have the capacity to stretch—but to a finite degree. Successful people are busy for a reason: They are remarkably good at what they do and almost always accomplish their goals. They've developed systems, processes, and accountability metrics to keep them on track. As a result, many ideal mentors are stretched to their capacity with their own professional and personal commitments. Having a mentoring team distributes the workload and responsibilities and mitigates the risk of neglecting other necessary responsibilities or, even worse, burning out.

- **Both parties gain a safety net for unforeseen circumstances:** Today's workforce is more transient than previous generations. Any number of reasons from personal to professional may influence a mentor's decision to leave their job or organization. In a mentorship dyad, your departure could leave your mentee abandoned in a way that may damage not only their learning but possibly their future career path. Conversely, you may have invested resources and time into a mentee—only to have them depart for personal or professional reasons. This leaves you, as mentor, conflicted. On the one hand, you may be elated to see your mentee leave for a better opportunity. On the flip side, you may also be upset that another organization is now the beneficiary of the countless hours spent developing a rising star.

  The good news is that mentoring can be virtual and does not need to be extinguished just because the mentor or mentee departed. It will, however, look and feel different. We will discuss this in greater depth in Chapter 6.

What's more, a team of mentors helps protect against mentorship malpractice[3]—toxic mentor behaviors that jeopardize a mentee's chance of success (discussed in Chapter 4). Mentoring teams may actually help the mentor grow their professional network with other members of the team, especially those outside their field. For example, a medical school faculty member mentoring someone with a nursing background can now develop relationships with and collaborate with an entirely different specialty as they engage with someone through a mentoring committee. A mentor can also learn different mentoring styles and approaches from the other mentors on the team that they can then apply to future mentees.

What's important to understand is that the mentee should have multiple mentors and that they don't all need to know one another. The mentee should pollinate these relationships and reach out to the mentor who is best suited to help the mentee with a particular task or challenge.

Step 2. Initiate a Trial Run

You don't need to get along with everyone. As early as preschool, you realize that you gravitate toward some people and others not so much. This basic human dynamic must be considered before any mentoring relationship is created. For a mentoring relationship to be fruitful, it needs to have all-around good "chemistry." It's not just about matching personality types (which has been debunked[4]) or how much someone "likes" another person. It's about finding the right fit in terms of values, work ethic, expectations, knowledge, and temperament. It's about the shared vision of success and the timeline to get there. Ultimately, as a mentor you must have and be willing to share the knowledge and, when appropriate, members of your network—your social capital.

Contrary to popular belief, 61% of mentoring relationships happen organically.[5] There is usually no formal matching system. People simply gravitate toward those they know, like, and trust. They also see in potential mentors what they wish to become themselves. Yet in some cases, assigned mentors are necessary for moving through residency, PhD committees, and similar academic journeys.

Fair warning: Watch out for possible "implicit bias." Could your negative reaction to the mentee or mentor stem from the fact that they don't look, think, or act like you? Our brains rely on mental shortcuts, known as heuristics, that can kick in automatically. Mentoring across differences is discussed more in Chapter 5. By staying mindful (discussed more fully in Chapter 15), you can guard against this common human tendency and build more meaningful connections.

Before agreeing to mentor anyone, give careful thought to the person who will be your mentee. Remember, you'll be sacrificing your professional time and energy to help this person succeed. This decision should not be taken lightly.

The best mentees are diamonds in the rough. They have the raw talent and potential but need someone to guide them, show them "pro tips," and give them reasonable targets to reach. Look for someone who has demonstrated they are ambitious and organized, while simultaneously independent and flexible. Many mentor–mentee relationships have soured because a mentee couldn't problem solve on their own or harassed their mentor with innumerable questions which could easily have been Googled.[6] Others have failed because communication became one-sided, feedback was met with furiosity not curiosity, or one person wasn't tolerant of perspectives that differed from their own. See Chapter 9 for further "mentee landmines."

Perhaps most importantly, ask yourself: Do I *trust* this person? Whether maintaining the integrity of private and confidential discussions, concerns over scientific conduct, or authorship, the mentor should never take on a mentee they cannot learn to trust. (The converse is obviously true as well.) Though thankfully rare, several examples exist of mentors and mentees who have committed academic fraud, thereby jeopardizing both of their careers.

So how does one choose the right protégé? Selecting the right mentee may be as simple as doing a "trial run" before you commit. Consider one of the following approaches to ensure alignment before you commit to mentorship.

The Reading Test

Most people are not willing to do the work. Tell your prospective mentee to read a book or journal article from your field that you find particularly influential. Ask them to set up another meeting in a month's time, and before that meeting, ask them to share a written sample of their thoughts. Our experience is that most potential mentees will never be heard from again.

If a mentee is willing to invest the time in reading, interpreting, and reviewing the paper with you, you know that the mentee is hungry and committed to growth. The discussion also serves as an opportunity to listen to their ideas and decipher whether they have the knowledge, passion, and initiative needed to advance with limited guard rails.

If they don't make that follow-up appointment or show up with incoherent or poorly prepared responses, you have likely saved yourself from a time-consuming and potentially unhelpful mentoring relationship. Be especially wary of potential mentees who are always armed with excuses. To paraphrase Benjamin Franklin, "Show me someone who is very good at excuses, and I will show you someone very good at little else."

The Writing Assignment

American author David McCullough said, "Writing is thinking. To write well is to think clearly. That's why it's so hard." Even when one doesn't feel it's their strength, a writing exercise is a good way to assess a prospective mentee's thought process and analysis. It also helps demonstrate a mentee's willingness to learn and how open they are to feedback—do they see it as a criticism or opportunity for growth?

As part of the reading test or as a separate check, ask a prospective mentee to share a writing sample or to pen a synopsis of a key article in their field.

A one- or two-pager is sufficient. Give them a reasonable deadline with expectations around content and word count so they know what you expect.

Like the book test, the writing assignment offers unique insights into the prospective mentee's ideas, thought processes, and philosophies. It also helps determine whether they can "get over the goal line"—someone who finishes what they start.

On-the-Job Test Run

In the management world, it is not uncommon to take a mentee on a sales call or to a client meeting. In healthcare, you can have the mentee attend a research meeting or stakeholder convention. A debrief, or after-action review, with your mentee after such a meeting can be an additional opportunity to assess their readiness to embark on this growth journey.

Much as you would do at a morbidity and mortality conference, review with your potential mentee their impressions, analysis, and changes they would make based on what you both saw. This gives you both a chance not just to experience the opportunity but to collectively reflect on it. If your mentee puts in a sincere effort and demonstrates curiosity and competency during the "test," this is a positive sign that you can move forward. It also gives you a sense of how they think on their feet—a key component of creativity and future success.

Gain Collateral Information

Your prospective mentee undoubtedly looked you up and searched the web for information about your expertise, interests, and accomplishments. There's a good chance they also reached out to former mentees. In addition to these tests and your own "gut instinct," you should also gather information on the mentee. It usually begins by asking the mentee for their curriculum vitae (CV) (if it is in an academic setting) or resume. See if they have first-authored papers or chapters, taken on leadership roles, or have experience conducting research projects. It is also helpful to see where they went to school and what their hobbies are—topics you may want to bring up when first meeting them to forge a connection. While formal letters of recommendation are over the top, reaching out informally to people they formerly worked with for a conversation might shed some light on capabilities and opportunities for growth. It is also a good idea to have them meet some of your current mentees (those you trust) to assess what they think about this person's abilities and potential.

Consider a mentee who is a physician in training (usually referred to as a "house officer," "resident," or subspecialty "fellow"). We would ask those who worked most closely with them in the clinical setting—such as their supervising attending, residency director, nursing staff, social workers—what they were like in a team setting. Some questions to consider are:

1. What was their knowledge level or performance on in-training exams?
2. Did they return pages from nurses in a timely manner?
3. When asked to do so, did they come to evaluate unstable patients at the bedside?
4. Were they hardworking? Thoughtful? Kind? Can you think of an example?
5. Did they get along well with colleagues? Were they liked by the other members of their cohort?
6. Were there any red—or even yellow—flags in terms of ethical behavior?
7. Would you want them to care for your family member?

We do the same when we hire faculty. For example, for job candidates, we ask the administrative staff who escorts them what their thoughts are on the candidate. Some of us even include the drivers who escort them around for appointments to get a sense of their interactions. People often let their guard down and show their true colors in front of someone they feel has no sway in the decision-making process. Generally, those who "kiss up" often "kick down." Indeed, the person presumably lowest on the organizational ladder will often get a remarkably accurate sense of what someone is really like.

Of course, one negative comment should not derail things, but you'd be surprised how often behavioral patterns emerge. You need to consider whether they are someone whom you want to entrust with your reputation. At this point, you may question if choosing a mentee needs to be this difficult and time-consuming? The answer is "no," provided you are fine with spending time on a mentoring relationship gone awry. As the saying goes, "Measure twice, cut once." If you put the work in on the front end, you will have fewer time-consuming catastrophes to deal with on the back end. And perhaps more importantly, putting in the effort now may avoid failed relationships that don't just take up time but also reduce your desire to mentor in the future.

A working relationship with a mentee can last a lifetime but shouldn't feel like a life sentence. Best to choose wisely.

Step 3. Make a Game Plan

As with any relationship, the key to success is open communication and having compatible goals and expectations. The same goes for mentees. Once you've selected your mentee, establish ground rules so that you both feel you are growing and benefiting from the relationship. This is critical to making communication and interactions both positive and efficient. While we will dive into this further in other chapters, at minimum, your discussion should establish:

- **Your mentee's short- and long-term goals:** These should be revisited regularly since people's goals may (and should) evolve over time.

- **A regular meeting schedule, time, and place to cover progress, roadblocks, and questions:** How do you want to handle issues that arise between the set meeting times?

- **What constitutes an urgent matter:** Urgent matters should not wait until your regular meeting (but unscheduled meetings are best kept to a minimum).

- **What services you will provide to your mentee (and, conversely, what you will not):** For example, if your mentee wants to finish a paper or project, you will provide your services to ensure that gets done. Within this work, you may agree to provide some analytical support, time at the bench to complete experiments, access to data sources, citation management from a research associate in your group, etc. These types of details are important to go over so that misunderstandings do not occur.

- **Your expectations of your mentee:** Expectations may be regarding professional behavior, work quality, and specific milestones they should accomplish. Let them know what "excellent" looks like.

- **The tone and expectations when dealing with mistakes and problems:** You don't expect perfection (mentees are still learning, and we're all human, after all), but you do expect honesty as well as a willingness to work on finding solutions. When mistakes occur or your mentee encounters challenges, they should be upfront, timely, and have a plan to deal with it—or at least the outline of a plan.

The foundation of a successful mentoring relationship lies in trust for both parties. It should be a safe and confidential zone for discussing aspects that might be sensitive in nature. Bottom line, your mentee should never hesitate to bring these issues to your attention. In turn, you, as the mentor, should feel comfortable providing candid feedback with the assumption that such information will be accepted as an opportunity to reflect, learn, and grow.

Mentoring relationships work best when there is a defined time to meet, and the topic of discussion is known in advance. New mentoring relationships often benefit from regular meetings every two to four weeks. The mentee should prepare an agenda; provide status updates on projects, current needs, or challenges; and state what questions or discussion points they would like to cover during the face-to-face time. Depending on the urgency and complexity of current needs, other items can be trimmed or modified to allow for a rich discussion. So that you can prepare for the meeting and add or modify items if needed, ask for the agenda and any pre-reads in advance. The agenda does not need to be formal; an email will suffice. There are different formats for an agenda, so don't be overly wed to just one approach. Boxes 1.1 and 1.2 outline a couple of different formats. For example, for longer mentoring meetings or for meeting with your mentorship team as a whole, Box 1.2 may serve as a good example, whereas for shorter meetings, Box 1.1 may work well. But, remember, asking for an agenda or materials means you, as mentor, must also come prepared to the meeting.

Box 1.1 Example Mentoring Agenda 1

Date: [Insert Date]
Time: [Insert Start and End Time]

1. **Review of Previous Action Items (5 minutes)**

   - Discuss progress on tasks since last meeting.
   - Address any challenges faced in completing these tasks.

2. **Current Topics for Discussion (10 minutes)**

   - [Topic 1: Description]
   - [Topic 2: Description]

3. **Feedback and Guidance (5 minutes)**

   - Mentor provides feedback on recent work or specific projects.
   - Mentee shares any concerns or areas where they seek guidance.

4. **Review of Goals and Planning (5 minutes)**

   - Review goals, and ensure work is still in alignment.
   - Identify resources or support needed to achieve these goals.

5. **Next Steps and Action Items (5 minutes)**

   - Summarize agreed-upon tasks and responsibilities.
   - Establish completion dates and follow-up timeline.

Box 1.2 Example Mentoring Agenda 2

I. **Goals**

  a. Short-term (within 1 year)

    i. Create a series of teaching scripts.

    ii. Fully establish Monday morning telehealth clinic.

    iii. Create/improve electronic database for transplant patients.

  b. Mid-term (2–3 years)

    i. Enhance fellows' and residents' experience in clinic/rotation.

    ii. Learn how to help medical students improve their notes and presentations.

    iii. Create policies on typical practices and common conditions in our clinic.

  c. Long-term (> 3–5 years)

    i. Continue with research opportunities especially focusing on quality improvement and patient safety projects.

    ii. Go up for promotion to full professor in the clinical track.

II. **Assessment of Satisfaction with Current Role and Responsibilities**

  a. Satisfied with the difference I've been able to make in the patients I've assumed care for in clinic.

  b. Will be taking over additional clinical duties so I would like to discuss with the committee what my priorities should be given increased workload.

  c. I am having some issues related to nursing support that I need guidance on.

III. **Education**

  a. Fellows' evaluations

    i. 4.5 to 4.7 (out of 5) in the categories

    ii. "Provided independence with great oversight . . . great bedside manner"

    iii. "Thoughtful in her approach toward supervising and teaching fellows while still allowing the fellow full autonomy"

b. Residents' evaluations

   i. 4.7 to 4.9 in the categories

   ii. "Knowledgeable," "approachable," "encourages discussion," "great teacher"

   iii. "Felt supported," "allowed autonomy," "wonderful patient rapport and great role model for patient interactions"

   iv. Areas for improvement: "provide educational chalk talks," "5–10-minute didactics would be great on consults"

c. Self-appraisal

   i. I enjoy both my clinics and attending on general medicine. I would like to discuss how I can address some of the evaluations from learners.

IV. **Clinical Work**

a. Making sure patients are getting their follow-up appointments

b. I am having difficulty keeping up with both inpatient and outpatient issues

V. **Scholarly Activity**

a. Two first-authored papers that are currently accepted

b. Collaborative effort paper ("I am 3rd author") about to be submitted

c. Goal is to publish 2–4 peer-reviewed papers per year: "I am on track"

VI. **Leadership Roles**

a. Clinic—working to establish relationship with nursing leaders

b. Fellowship—running/organizing orientation and re-orienting fellows as needed

Finally, remember, this is your reputation on the line. Be explicit on defining what constitutes egregious errors and how these will be handled. Plagiarism, scientific misconduct, abusive conduct, and the like are grounds to terminate the relationship and may result in disciplinary action. If the mentee is made aware of this up-front, there can be no question later about the consequences, should these unfortunate issues arise. No, you don't need a signed contract. But yes, please strongly consider having this discussion.

Summary

Effective mentorship requires careful planning and forethought before jumping in. As Benjamin Franklin said, "An ounce of prevention is worth a pound of cure." Although selecting the right mentee and setting clear expectations may require significant time and effort initially, these steps can prevent future stress and complications.

Starting a mentoring relationship on a solid foundation benefits both parties, making it a mutually rewarding experience. If you're unsure where to start in your new role as "mentor," consider a trial run with your mentee. Assigning a reading or writing task can be telling when evaluating how dedicated and driven your prospective mentee is. While preparation is key, remember that not all of the pressure is on you. Encouraging a mentee to establish a team of mentors works toward their benefit and yours.

Take-Home Points

- If asked to mentor someone, evaluate their work ethic, drive, organization, and communication skills. Determine whether they are willing to put in the work to help themselves get the most out of a mentoring relationship.
- Put in time and effort prior to starting your mentorship relationship to lay the groundwork. Setting clear expectations regarding meeting cadence, goals, time commitment, and communication will benefit both mentor and mentee.
- Establish a mentoring team. This relieves a sole mentor from having to "do it all" and allows the mentee the opportunity to learn from people with a variety of experiences and backgrounds.

2

Know Your Role

One of Vineet's mentees reached out for help on how to develop a protocol for a systematic review. Another asked Sanjay for a letter of support for a grant application. And a third wanted to connect with Ruth to talk about how to approach job interviews and how to expand their professional network.

When it comes to mentorship, one size does not fit all. It doesn't even fit many. Each person is unique and requires bespoke mentoring approaches, supports, and challenges to get ahead. The mentor has a repertoire of experiences, a broad network, strengths they can rely on, and challenges they've learned from. Each also has a different identity and upbringing; drawing on these experiences is what strengthens their mentoring. Mentees benefit from various types of mentors and would benefit from the diversity of experiences and perspectives.

By recognizing your strengths as a mentor and the needs of your mentee, you can leverage your abilities to ensure your protégé's success. As shown in Figure 2.1, there are at least four distinct mentoring archetypes and roles to consider when approaching mentees.[1]

The Traditional Mentor

The traditional (or career) mentor is invested in the long-term growth of a mentee. Traditional mentors are in it for the duration of the mentoring journey. Some consider these types of mentors their "career mentor"—someone the mentee can turn to with nearly any kind of question or dilemma. The job of the traditional mentor is to support and encourage the mentee, open doors they never knew existed, and help the mentee form

DOI: 10.1201/9781003611233-3

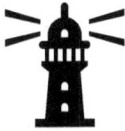

MENTOR

Guides from experience

- Shares wisdom from years of clinical or research practice
- Helps you navigate career choices and professional dilemmas
- Offers a long-term partnership focused on growth and leadership

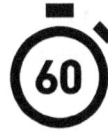

COACH

Develops targeted skills

- Focuses on specific skills (e.g., time and conflict management, executive presence)
- Does not require experience in your domain or industry
- Brings valuable, actionable strategies to individuals and groups of mentees

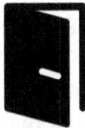

SPONSOR

Opens doors to opportunity

- Actively advocates for promotions, grants, and leadership roles
- Uses their social or political capital to advance your career
- Speaks your name in rooms where decisions are made

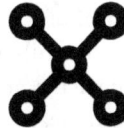

CONNECTOR

Curates introductions for growth

- Taps into a well-developed network to make thoughtful, strategic introductions
- Helps you meet potential mentors, coaches, and sponsors
- Builds authentic relationships rather than accumulating contacts

FIGURE 2.1 Four common mentor archetypes.

a mentoring team or circle. They prepare them for the opportunities and help them succeed. They have a higher and longer view and can offer much needed perspective.

Traditionally, the mentor was older and more senior, but, as previously discussed, a mentoring team with diverse views and backgrounds and varying levels of experience[2] is the more contemporary and preferred approach.

The mentor meets regularly with the mentee to help them grow in their specific discipline. A primary mentor in healthcare is noted for their deep content or methodological knowledge—often in the same field as their mentee. They also have eminence and a network that they can harness for a mentee's benefit. Primary career mentors surround their mentee with additional colleagues to ensure the mentee's success.

In one way or another, for the duration of the mentee's career, your name will always be connected to theirs. They will often recognize you as the person who mentored them, or you will be known by the many things your mentee will accomplish. It's an enormous responsibility to mentor someone to those levels and is not to be taken lightly. The role requires attention to detail, helpful and targeted feedback, and a substantial investment of time to ensure the mentee is producing high-quality work and is on a path to success. Trust and respect are the necessary underpinnings of this type of mentoring relationship. Without them, the mentoring relationship will disintegrate.

The end goal of a traditional mentoring relationship is to ensure the mentee learns the skills and knowledge necessary to succeed on their own. In fact, in medicine and healthcare, that is how the success of the relationship is often measured. A traditional mentor is therefore a guide who will nurture and advocate for their mentee, much like a parent may for a child.

In North America, mentors are not traditionally paid. On occasion, they may get swag or a "thank you." Many organizations, however, require evidence of successful mentoring to reach the senior ranks of academia. But finances are never the motivating factor. Rather, altruism and a belief in ensuring the success of the field by passing on wisdom and paying forward that which someone else did for you are the hallmarks.

As the mentoring relationship evolves and stretches out over time, the mentor may (and should) learn from the mentee. Referred to as "reverse mentoring,"[3]— or reciprocal learning[4]—the mentee can serve as a mentor to the mentor (e.g., helping with social media or relatively new and highly technical methodological approaches). As mentees progress and develop their individual talents and skills, it may become difficult to tell who is the mentor and who is the mentee. The relationship becomes symbiotic and mutually beneficial.

The Coach

Ruth coached Dr. Zachary Turnbull, an anesthesiologist at Weill Cornell Medicine. His strong clinical skills, passion, and strong operations competency—complete with two master's degrees after his medical degree—led to his rise quickly through the ranks to a vice-chair role. While he knew how to do the work, he needed a confidential sounding board to help him prepare for politically charged conversations, workplace dynamics, and the delegation of tasks to his new staff. That's where the coaching came in. Once those skills were met, they went on to tackle new challenges.

Coaches usually work with a mentee for defined periods of time and focus their energy on improving a prespecified skillset. Examples may include how to manage conflict, build executive presence, improve time management, or delegate work. Coaches don't need to have experience in the mentee's domain or industry. Rather, they bring to a mentee a skill that is necessary for them to succeed.

Coaching does not involve the same investment of time, energy, or industry knowledge as traditional (or career) mentorship. It's a one-and-done type of deal. For example, Vineet had a tennis coach who focused purely on his serve. Didn't matter if he won or lost games, the key was to get the toss, weight, and contact point correct each and every time. Once he mastered it, that job was done. Sanjay had a more senior faculty member who was known as a great speaker coach him on his PowerPoint slides and presentation delivery. Those who have given TED talks have worked with a coach (or two) to ensure the talk is concise and impactful. Coaches therefore work with clients for a specified period of time, such as six months, and meet at a regular cadence. In healthcare, common examples of coaching-related engagements include strategy (such as negotiating job searches or contracts), a specific methodology (e.g., qualitative analysis), clinical skills (in the operating room[5] or on the wards[6]), or preparing a focused presentation. Coaches can also help define and refine your leadership style.

A coach can take on several different mentees at once due to the smaller time commitment. While informal coaches are not remunerated with money, formal coaches do get paid, and the good ones get paid well. For some, coaching may become their full-time career, and they are known as being exceptional in general or in specific areas (such as behavior change to impact leadership). They generally have a clear process and system to work with someone and often help the mentee work effectively with others. Like mentors, coaches expect their mentees to come ready and prepared to learn.

Coaching can be one-on-one or conducted in a small group when several people have the same challenges they'd like help in overcoming.[7] A coach's limited role means they are usually not a primary mentor for a particular mentee seeking their advice. However, primary mentors who become busier and may not be able to take on more mentees may focus on coaching a small number of individuals. In the mentoring ecosystem, coaches are integral contributors to a mentee's success and a vital element of their professional development.

The Sponsor

The sponsor talks about you (in a good way) when you're not in the room. While they don't generally provide advice or guidance as a traditional mentor or coach may, they use their sphere of influence—also known as their social or political capital[8]—in a field to help propel or aid a mentee. As a result, sponsors are typically higher up on the healthcare food chain (C-suite members, chiefs, chairs, or deans) and look to use their influence to support high-caliber people.

Sponsors can create opportunities and make them happen for the mentee by leveraging the network they've cultivated over the years. For example, sponsors may help their mentee land a spot on a national panel or be selected as a keynote speaker at a national society meeting. Sponsors could also help a mentee's career by writing a strong letter of recommendation for a job position or membership in an honorific society.

But it's not just what happens behind closed doors that counts as sponsorship. Social media are critical and often underutilized sponsorship tools. With one post, all of a sponsor's following are notified about the good work of the mentee. Dr. Kafui Dzirasa, a physician-scientist at Duke University School of Medicine, is sensational at doing this. Whenever one of his mentee's gets an NIH fellowship or publishes a paper, he takes a picture with them and posts it on his social media along with the congratulatory announcement. He unabashedly throws his support behind his mentees. It sends a strong signal to his followers that says, "I trained this person. They are fantastic and achieving great things. Keep an eye out for them because the best is yet to come."

Sponsors use their political capital to benefit the mentee and shine a light on them. In return, sponsors solidify their legacy as identifying, cultivating, and promoting "stars" and ensuring the success of their field.

It's for this last reason that we cautiously remind you to choose your mentees wisely. It's not just their reputation at risk; it's yours as well. It would behoove you to remind your mentees of this not inconsequential fact.

You've spent years, decades perhaps, developing your reputation. It doesn't take much for it to be threatened. We each have limited social and political capital. It's a finite resource and should be used wisely.

If you are going to serve as a sponsor, you want to select someone who has proven to be a worthy candidate and is willing to put in the work toward becoming successful. Beware of sponsoring someone who is struggling to find their stride and hoping you can wave a magic wand and make them successful. The mentee must do the work and achieve the accolades for you to brag about. So, before throwing your reputation behind a mentee, carefully evaluate their success potential using both objective metrics (such as publications, grants, previous accomplishments) and subjective feedback (from those with whom the mentee has worked). It's a careful mix of looking back, vis-à-vis their past accomplishments, and looking forward, via their potential.

Unfortunately, studies have shown that sponsorship is not equally distributed.[9–11] Women and members of certain underrepresented groups are far less likely to have someone advocate on their behalf or identify someone who acts as a sponsor. Lack of sponsorship may be partially to blame for the continued gap in leadership between the genders and other minority groups despite an increasing parity at entry-level positions[12] in many fields. A common adage for women in particular is that it is common to be over-mentored and under-sponsored.[13] Sponsors are human, and we tend to gravitate toward people who look like ourselves.[14] As a sponsor, be aware of this bias and take inventory of those whom you have traditionally sponsored. For example, how many are men or women, how many are from your organization versus others, and how many are in your field versus other, related domains? See if a pattern needs to be investigated, and recalibrate if needed. Be cognizant of whom you sponsor. After all, different perspectives increase creativity and lead to contributions that can be extremely valuable. You can learn from them as much as they learn from you.

As a sponsor, you don't necessarily need to broadcast that you've supported or recommended individuals for specific tasks. Some sponsorship is better done incognito. But a mentee may seek you out—and you should know what to look for and whether it's worth the risk!

The Connector

Many mentors have developed deep and well-curated networks. But having the network and being willing to make introductions to support a mentee are two separate things. Connectors have unique value. They are willing to tap into their well-developed network, often referred to as the golden Rolodex (by Generation X and earlier generations), or contact list (starting with Millennials), knowing exactly whom the mentee should talk to on a particular subject. They can introduce the mentee to a potential mentor, coach, or sponsor. They are expert networkers not because they collect contacts but rather because they develop key relationships over time. Connectors often know more than just a person's name and title. Rather, they can tell you about their hobbies, family, and last place they went on vacation. They have a magical ability to make people feel seen, and, when they talk to someone, they make them feel like the only person in the room. While they may not have the bandwidth or desire to mentor in the traditional sense, they are motivated by seeing the field and people succeed, and strongly believe in creating a nurturing pipeline for rising stars. They don't—or at least they shouldn't—absently introduce people, as, for instance, the sponsor; it is their reputation on the line. Rather, every connection is carefully curated and considered.

Connectors are pivotal conduits to mentees, mentors, and their field at large. In Malcom Gladwell's book, *The Tipping Point*, they are considered the hubs of social networks and literally serve as such.[15] For example, a connector helps mentees succeed by introducing them to potential mentors, sponsors, or coaches. Conversely, connectors help mentors by identifying prospective talent—those diamonds in the rough—or defining areas where coaching might be helpful, or people who would benefit from sponsorship. In making these introductions, connectors breathe life into their industry by helping ensure that their field continues to attract and retain the best, most effective, and influential people. In doing so, they are investing in the next generation of their well-curated network.

Where can you find connectors? In healthcare, these individuals are often in senior leadership roles and have acquaintances beyond their department and organization. They tend to be senior members of institutional and department leadership, such as department chairs and deans, board members, journal editors, or presidents. They are individuals who thrive on tapping into their extensive network to promote new people in the field. If you need a connector, ask your mentor and look up the organizational chart—you're likely to find a few there.

But fair warning: Don't overlook people just because they are less senior in the organization. Influence isn't just assigned; it's emergent. Many people are respected for their abilities regardless of their title and have developed deep networks as a result. Also, remember that social media have made it easier than ever to connect with people. Often, those who are junior have mastered the craft. They know how to directly reach out to CEOs, hospital directors, deans, and department chairs. Just attend your favorite national association meeting, and you will notice that some people simply seem to know everyone. They've never met a stranger, or so it seems. Breaking into these groups[16] may seem like a challenge, but it's not. If you can connect with one such "influencer," they will likely introduce you to others. They consider these introductions a badge of honor. That said, don't ask for an introduction the first time you meet someone. That sounds like a transaction. Instead, nurture the relationship and play the long game.

Summary

Four of the more common archetypes are the traditional (or career) mentor, the coach, the sponsor, and the connector. Each offers value to the mentee, but their roles do not look the same—each vary in their level and type of support of a mentee. Whether you are skilled at providing detailed feedback on a mentee's career path or are more comfortable talking someone up to highlight their accomplishments among those in higher-up positions, there's a role for you as a mentor. A well-rounded mentoring team will include one of each of these four mentor archetypes. At some point in your career, you may find yourself having filled all four of these roles, to the success of not only your mentees but the field as a whole.

Take-Home Points

- Traditional mentors invest in the long-term support of their mentee by guiding and supporting their career trajectory. This involves a substantial time commitment from the mentor; thus it may help to build a mentoring team.
- The coach offers expertise in a specific area or skillset that the mentee would like to grow in. This relationship may be shorter term, ending once the mentee has "mastered" what the coach has taught.
- Sponsors speak up for their mentees when they're not in the room. These individuals use their influence to recommend a mentee for select honors, awards, or speaking opportunities, helping the mentee be noticed in their field.
- Connectors have a so-called golden Rolodex or contact list. These individuals identify talent and use their deep and well-curated networks to make introductions that support a mentee. They may introduce mentees to potential collaborators, mentors, or sponsors.

3

Six Rules for Effective Mentoring

Mentoring, when done right, is intoxicating. But don't get drunk on the power. As Stan Lee once said of Spider Man, "With great power comes great responsibility." In healthcare, mentors wield power over their mentees because they have greater experience, eminence, and reputation. They are also in the role that can decide the future of the mentee. In medical school, they write letters of recommendation, and in residency, they determine performance on a rotation, both of which have significant implications. And as faculty, promotion is often hanging on the line. Mentors often have administrative or leadership roles as well, which gives them additional power relative to mentees. We're not saying it's right; we're just saying this happens (more about this in Chapter 4). In most cases, this power is used benevolently—for a mentee's benefit. We will discuss all of these issues in the chapters ahead.

Before we touch on effective mentoring, it's important to face the music. There might be times when there are conflicts of interest, and it's best to deal with the possibility head-on in a transparent fashion.

Dealing with Conflicts of Interest

It is not unusual for a mentor to wear various "hats" in an organization. In addition to being someone's mentor, they may serve as an executive within the organization. They may have a title such as director, chair, or dean. The "hat" a mentor wears during the conversation may influence the advice they provide the mentee. For example, there may be certain scenarios when the best interests of the department or organization may not align

DOI: 10.1201/9781003611233-4

with those of your mentee.[1] They might be looking for a raise, and there is an opportunity at a competing hospital that accomplishes exactly that. It might be right for the mentee, but as a leader at the organization, you know how difficult and expensive it is to replace a physician or any other healthcare worker. How are you going to advise this person? Our recommendation is to be thoughtful and transparent about which "hat" you are wearing. You might say something like: "I am now going to remove my mentor's hat and put on my chief/chair/dean hat and explain why I think you should consider staying . . . ."

Second, *don't hide the internal battle you are facing*. Be honest and let the mentee know you have a conflict of interest or are feeling conflicted. A simple sentence such as, "I am biased when it comes to this decision," goes a long way to affirming that your stance may not be neutral. Then call out the hat you are wearing and share your opinion given your conflict of interest (e.g., "I don't want to see you go"). Finally, try to give them advice as if no conflict existed (e.g., "It's a wonderful opportunity at a great place, and the salary bump is unlikely to happen here, so you should seriously think about this").

Ultimately, there are six tried-and-true best practices to ensure you become an effective mentor.

Rule 1. Give Credit to Your Mentee

Recognition should be given, not taken. Mentoring is not about recognition for you as the mentor. Rather, it's about celebrating your mentee's achievements and efforts. It goes without saying that you should look for every opportunity to praise and give them the credit they've earned.[2]

In healthcare, the traditional way of recognition is to share the achievement in person or at meetings (departmental or division meetings, journal clubs, etc.) with the shout-out about your mentee. Let those in attendance know what milestone was achieved, grant was awarded, or paper was published.

Hybrid work, Zoom meetings, and the rise in use of social media have allowed us to get creative in how we recognize mentees. Here are a few of our favorite ways of honoring our mentees, which you might wish to consider.

1. **Share it on social media:** Go to your mentee's presentation, take a picture of them at the podium, and put out a congratulatory comment on your social media platforms mentioning—and tagging—them.

2. **Send a communication update:** Send an email to the department chair, senior leaders in your institution, and colleagues lauding the award that your mentee received or their accomplishment. Attach a photo of the mentee with the award or a link to the paper as an extra way of allowing your leaders to see the praise themselves. This brings the mentee's accomplishment front and center and informs those who may not have known about the mentee's accomplishment.

3. **Nominate your mentee for an award or recognition program:** Identify opportunities where your mentee and their work can shine, such as internal awards, national committees, or leadership development programs. Taking the time to write a thoughtful nomination not only elevates your mentee but also signals to others that you believe in their potential and contributions. It allows the mentee's name to be discussed in groups that have never heard of them and they otherwise may not have access to. Even if they don't win, the nomination itself is a powerful gesture that shows your commitment to their success. We often share nomination letters (especially if there isn't a positive outcome) with our mentees—it is a powerful way to actively show them your advocacy and belief in their abilities.

The humblebrag—that fine line between letting people know of your accomplishments and not sounding narcissistic—is challenging for even the most seasoned healthcare workers. It's almost impossible for those who are starting out. If the mentor publicly recognizes the accomplishments of the mentee, this alleviates that pressure (which for the mentee might feel like a burden) so they do not feel compelled to brag about themselves. After all, a competent, successful mentee reflects positively on you as well.

Rule 2. Give Your Mentee Duties That Benefit Their Growth, Not Yours

A mentee is not your personal assistant. They are not there to manage your projects or to tackle your to-do list. Any assignments you give to your mentee and any task that they take on independently should be to benefit their career, not yours.

This doesn't mean they can't work on projects that are of interest to you or those where you are the leader. Rather, you should both be excited about the project. Each project should be an opportunity for the mentee to grow and learn something, even if the education is not immediately apparent to them. But remember, just because you offer a project to them, it doesn't mean they should take it. One of the responsibilities of a mentor is to help

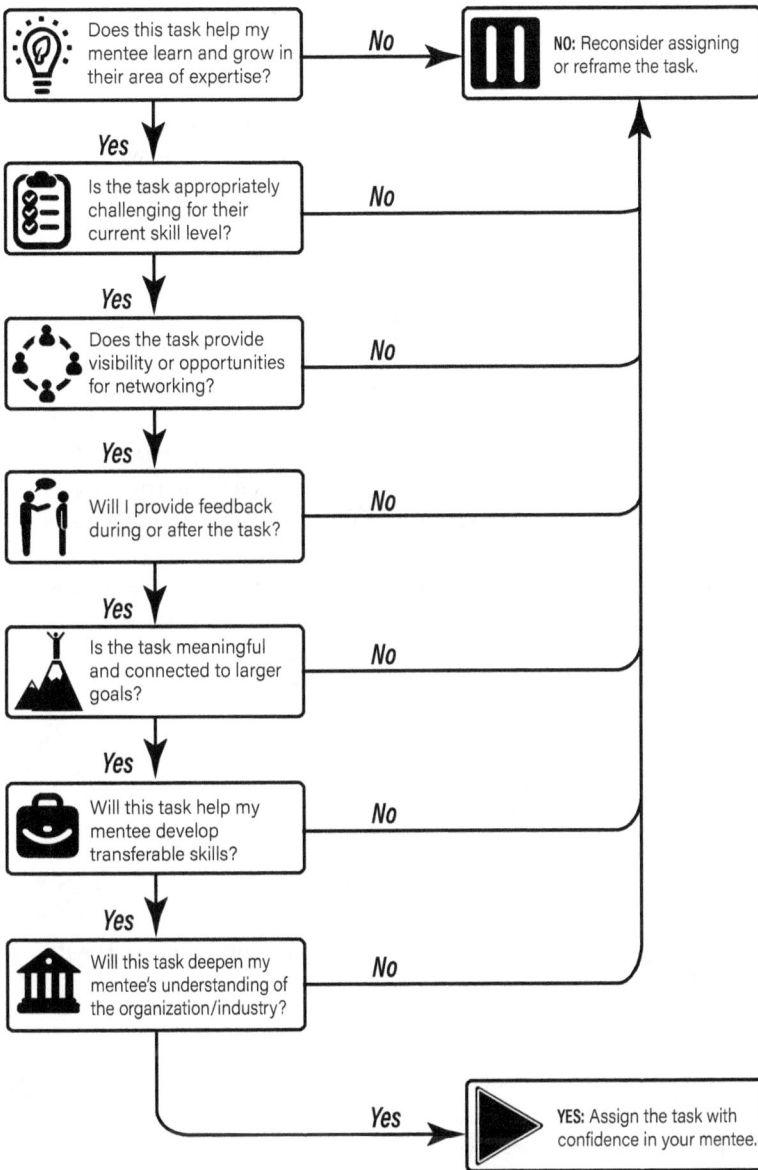

Does this task help my mentee learn and grow in their area of expertise? — **No** → **NO:** Reconsider assigning or reframe the task.

Yes ↓

Is the task appropriately challenging for their current skill level? — **No**

Yes ↓

Does the task provide visibility or opportunities for networking? — **No**

Yes ↓

Will I provide feedback during or after the task? — **No**

Yes ↓

Is the task meaningful and connected to larger goals? — **No**

Yes ↓

Will this task help my mentee develop transferable skills? — **No**

Yes ↓

Will this task deepen my mentee's understanding of the organization/industry? — **No**

Yes → **YES:** Assign the task with confidence in your mentee.

FIGURE 3.1 Decision algorithm for assigning a task to your mentee.

the mentee differentiate between a good project and one that is of interest to them—ideally, it's both. Resist pressuring them to do something—it is only short-term gain that usually leads to long-term pain. This type of issue is discussed in more detail in Chapter 4. Figure 3.1 displays a handy algorithm to use when thinking about assigning a task to your mentee.

Rule 3. Allow Your Mentee to Branch Out

In Chapter 1, we underscore the importance of a team of mentors and how leveraging a variety of perspectives benefits the mentees. But not all mentors are created equal. Some mentors—especially those who are insecure—prefer not sharing mentees.[3] (We'll talk more about this in Chapter 4.) Instead, they tend to lure their mentee (either deliberately or inadvertently) into an "exclusive relationship," isolating and preventing them from seeking guidance or collaborations with others. This is not only unethical and morally questionable but also likely to be unproductive for you as a mentor.

First, it stifles your mentee's development and their ability to learn a variety of approaches, styles, and strategies from others. Second, it makes the mentee reliant on you for everything—often leading to a significant volume of communication and meetings. Finally, it limits your opportunity to learn from the cross-pollination of knowledge from other experts in the mentee's field.

Don't sabotage your mentee's growth by being possessive. Encourage your mentee to expand their horizons, take risks, and connect with others. At the very least, it will save you time. Best case scenario: You and your mentee grow.

Rule 4. Keep Things Moving

Academic medicine has predictable milestones, such as medical school graduation, residency, fellowship, and rising through the ranks as faculty. But it's hard to get through each phase on your own, let alone prepare for the next one. To ensure your mentee is successful, meetings with a regular cadence must be scheduled.

As the mentor, you must have the bandwidth and desire to meet regularly with your mentee, answer their questions, and ensure their projects are moving forward. There are only 24 hours in the day, and if you are going to add a mentee, you will need to sacrifice something else. Choose wisely. Working longer hours and sleeping less is not a long-term solution. The most efficient mentors know how to run a "tight ship." For example, Vineet will often meet with mentees during travel if they are both going to the same scientific meeting. Sanjay blocks specific times of the week for mentoring activities, ensuring that they don't get eaten up by other tasks. And Ruth uses her commuting time for mentorship discussions.

At times, your mentee will seek your approval for a paper, grant, or professional interaction. Be sure you get back with them in a timely manner. Ghosting them (where your communication disappears for a period of time) or making your mentee follow-up with you multiple times for an answer will negatively impact the mentee and also your reputation as mentor. Mentors who insist on being engaged at every step but make mentees wait for several days or even weeks for a response become an obstacle to success. Don't become a bottleneck in your mentee's career progression.

It is important to remember that the mentee's timeline is usually different from yours. Simply put, it is usually shorter. You are already established and are a known entity. On the other hand, your mentee must prove themselves and often must do so relatively quickly (e.g., during their start-up period). This is especially true for looming deadlines like grant submissions, major presentations, or award nominations. Good mentors should seek to accelerate, not slow down success.

Rule 5. Embrace Difficult or Awkward Conversations

We're human. We don't always get along. The close relationship between a mentor and mentee means some disagreements are inevitable. It's not a question of whether they will happen, rather when. But if you can expect them, you can be better prepared to manage them with grace.

If you and your mentee share the goal of setting them up for success, they should be seeking your feedback.[4] They will also understand that, if you need to discuss sensitive issues with them, they must be managed with trust. If you are professional and set a goal of an honest resolution, even the stickiest of conversations can be resolved elegantly.

A mentor is not a parent, nor are they really a friend. (But as the relationship evolves over time, a friendship may develop.) So, while it may feel natural, don't try to be either of those. Rather, be calm, objective, and direct. If your mentee made a critical error, don't dwell on the past but focus on the future. Indeed, during times of crisis, next steps can be defining moments. Be clear about why an issue is a problem and what must happen to correct the situation. As well, be explicit about the timeline in which this should happen. A mentee should never be left uncertain as to what they should do when something goes awry. A little preparation and honesty go a long way to ensure a mistake becomes a teaching moment.

We have all had these discussions with our mentors, and we know that they are never easy. But we know how good mentors manage them. They have these discussions privately. They distinguish the person from the issue. They thank the mentee for their honesty in bringing the mistake to light. They offer clear guidance and assistance. And they reinforce their belief in a mentee's character and abilities. After all, candor without kindness amounts to cruelty.

Sometimes, it is best to take a pause. It's likely been a few years since you've been a resident, junior faculty member, or whatever stage your mentee is in. Before meeting with your mentee, try and remember what it was like for you at that stage—trying to impress those senior to you to get a recommendation letter or job offer, working long hours, missing lots of sleep, neglecting family gatherings due to your on-call schedule, and always feeling like you are not studying enough. Putting yourself in your mentee's shoes before and during the conversation will increase your self-awareness and empathy when you speak to your mentee. It will remind you that they are doing the best they can, under the circumstances, and will likely take the sting out of your tone.[5] We'll go much deeper into this idea in Chapter 15.

Rule 6. Be Available

Success snowballs, but time does not. The paradox about success is that as the mentor gets more of it, their ability to engage in the work that made them successful becomes limited. Have a scientific breakthrough, a landmark article, or a major award, and you suddenly find yourself caught in a whirlwind of meetings, speaking engagements, and travel that dominates your time. Such a demanding schedule can be an obstacle to fulfilling your duties as a mentor. But there are workarounds:

- **Try shorter meetings:** Who says all mentor meetings must last a full hour? If you can get to the heart of an issue in 30 minutes (or, occasionally, 20 minutes), make the meetings shorter! Parkinson's Law[6] states that work expands to fill the time. It's why we work better under looming deadlines or why we procrastinate till the very last minute. So make your meetings shorter. Shorter time blocks can teach your mentee strong communication skills as they are forced to get to their key concerns immediately, and you are forced to be concise in your response. Vineet's standard is now 30-minute monthly meetings with mentees. He focuses on three issues; each issue has ten minutes: five to summarize and five to discuss. Holding these types of meetings, however, requires an agenda and goal setting by the mentee. It also often requires pre-reading(s) by the mentor. In other words, both come prepared to make the most use of their time. Try it: It could be good for both of you!

- **Be creative:** Simple touchpoints can be just as helpful as longer mentoring meetings. A quick phone call on the weekend during a walk, a text message while you are waiting in line at Costco, or a brief email when it's least expected can help a mentee stay on track while allowing you to get other things done during the day. It's also a nice way to remind them you care and are thinking about them even beyond your usual sessions.

- **Technology is your friend:** Just because you are in a different time zone or hemisphere does not mean you cannot communicate. Some might argue that they communicate more efficiently. Use video conferencing such as Zoom or Teams and applications such as WhatsApp or Slack to your advantage. If you are traveling with your mentee, use travel time to your advantage. We've each had mentoring sessions at 30,000 feet, in an airport lounge, and in Ubers! It's uninterrupted time, which is golden.

- **Be realistic:** We're all busy. Decide whether your hectic life truly allows the time and the mental and emotional energy required to mentor someone effectively. A mentee will rely on your expertise—and your presence—on a regular basis. If you have intense travel or a grant deadline coming up, let your mentee know in advance that you are facing a crunch time and will have limited availability. This will allow them to plan accordingly.

Figure 3.2 summarizes these rules. Most importantly, don't overlook this critical component: Be present and fully engaged when you're with your mentee regardless of what else may be going on. Just because you *can* speak with your mentee (in person, over the phone, or via Zoom or Teams) does not mean that you are actually *communicating* in a meaningful or effective manner. This is particularly important if you find yourself distracted during the conversation (perhaps you are suddenly overwhelmed by all the tasks that are piling up) or trying to multitask (by simultaneously checking your emails) while putatively providing guidance to someone who is in need of your wisdom. This also holds during routine in-person encounters with your mentee: Fully engage by showing them that for the next 30 minutes they are all that matters. Put your computer and phone away. If you are with your mentee, be there fully. We discuss the importance of using mindfulness in a mentoring relationship in Chapter 15.

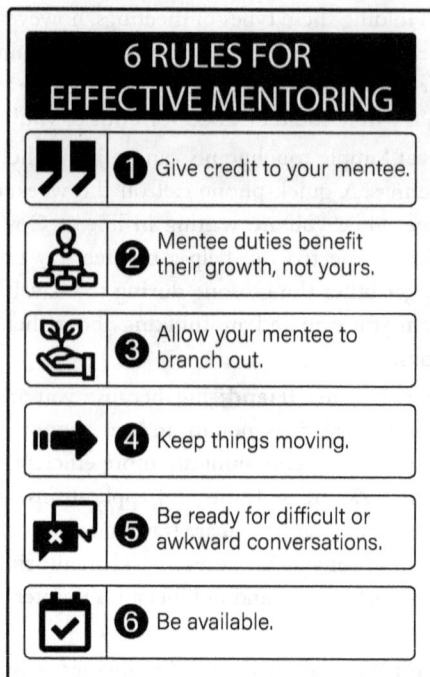

6 RULES FOR EFFECTIVE MENTORING

1. Give credit to your mentee.
2. Mentee duties benefit their growth, not yours.
3. Allow your mentee to branch out.
4. Keep things moving.
5. Be ready for difficult or awkward conversations.
6. Be available.

FIGURE 3.2 Six rules for effective mentoring.

Summary

Being a mentor goes beyond simply holding a title; it requires a genuine commitment to benevolence, self-reflection, and self-improvement, along with a keen awareness of power dynamics, especially in healthcare. Due to their experience and roles, mentors wield considerable influence, which can significantly impact a mentee's future through recommendations or evaluations. When conflicts of interest arise—such as a promising mentee considering leaving your organization—meet them with transparency and honesty. This necessitates being fully present with your mentee, no matter when or where those meetings occur.

Following these six rules of effective mentoring will help ensure that your mentorship is not only advantageous for the mentee but fulfilling for you as a mentor. Despite the investment of time, careful thought, and difficult conversations that mentorship entails, you have a wonderful opportunity to shape another professional, and their future mentees as well. When mentorship is done well, the rewards are tenfold.

Take-Home Points

- Effective mentoring involves conscious effort to put your mentee in the limelight, offer opportunities to benefit their growth, and assist them in expanding their network. You can accelerate their growth—don't stunt it by making them your personal assistant.

- Be ready to address difficult conversations in mentorship, whether it's managing personal conflicting interests, addressing critical errors, or talking through disagreements. Speak in kindness while bringing issues to light and reinforce your belief in the mentee's character and abilities.

- Be present in the moment. Dedicate your full attention to the conversation when you meet. If time is an issue, try shorter meetings! But don't sacrifice the quality of your time together—a mentee is in need of your guidance, after all.

4

Mentorship Malpractice: From Mentor to Tormentor

Every few years, *Nature*, a premiere scientific journal, runs a survey of graduate students to get a litmus test of how they think their training is progressing.[1] In 2022, over 3,000 students responded to the survey.[2] And what they had to say about the state of mentorship at their institution was not good . . . at all.

More than one-fifth of the students (22%) stated that if they could start things all over again, they would have changed supervisors—the principal mentor for a graduate student. Sadly, this statistic shows little improvement since the 2019 survey. Furthermore, more than a quarter of the survey respondents (26%) indicated they would change their institution, revealing potentially toxic work environments. One student commented, "Supervisor/lab group is everything. Topic/field doesn't matter. The environment you work in is most important to help you get through the graduate degree."[2] The National Academies of Sciences, Engineering and Medicine report on the Science of Effective Mentoring in STEMM (science, technology, engineering, mathematics, and medicine) reported that a positive mentoring relationship is the "most important factor in completing a STEMM degree."[3] At a time when we are hemorrhaging healthcare workers and scientists, could we be our own worst enemy?

So what leads to this severe dissatisfaction, which is causing a mass exodus from our healthcare system? Simply put, these terrible, horrible, no good, very bad mentors are colloquially (and not affectionately) called *tormentor mentors*.[4] The actions engaged in are what we call *mentorship malpractice*.[5]

Mentorship malpractice falls into two buckets based on the behavior—active and passive. Active mentorship malpractice can be easily identified

DOI: 10.1201/9781003611233-5

by dysfunctional behavior that is overt, blatant, and easily recognizable. When you hear about the behavior, your pulse quickens, eyebrows shoot up, and eyes widen. It's the kind of stuff that makes you cringe.

Passive mentorship malpractice, on the other hand, is more covert, insidious, and identifiable by inaction. Here, your eyebrows may scrunch in confusion. Is it truly bad behavior, or are there other perfectly good reasons for why this may have happened?

Mentorship in healthcare is not just about career guidance—it directly impacts patient care, professional development, and the overall culture of medical institutions. When mentorship is effective, it fosters skilled, confident, productive, and ethical professionals who provide high-quality care. But when mentorship turns toxic—when it crosses into mentorship malpractice—the consequences extend far beyond individual careers.

Poor mentorship can contribute to burnout,[6] erode trust, decrease psychological safety,[7] and perpetuate a dysfunctional culture that stifles innovation and collaboration. In a field where decisions can mean the difference between life and death, the presence of tormentor mentors and their destructive influence can reverberate throughout entire healthcare systems, affecting both healthcare providers and patients alike.

This is why identifying and addressing both is paramount. The overt and shocking behaviors of active mentorship malpractice may be easier to spot, but the quiet, insidious nature of passive malpractice—where opportunities for guidance, advocacy, and development are neglected—can be just as damaging. In either case, the result is a breakdown in the mentorship ecosystem, leading to dissatisfaction, disillusionment, and ultimately the loss of talented professionals from the field.

Ultimately, bad mentoring is worse than no mentoring.[8] Once a mentee has been on the receiving end of toxic mentoring, they are likely not going to want to dip their toe in the mentoring pool again. That's unfortunate as they will miss out on the plethora of mentoring benefits, including higher salaries, increased promotions, lower burnout, more publications, protected research time, and higher self-efficacy.[9,10] Understanding and addressing mentorship malpractice is therefore not just an ethical imperative—it is a strategic necessity for the sustainability and effectiveness of our healthcare workforce. Figure 4.1 presents six common types of mentorship malpractice—three active, three passive—and each is damaging in its own way. For strategies mentees can employ to navigate troubled mentorship, see Chapter 10.

6 TYPES OF
MENTORSHIP MALPRACTICE

ACTIVE

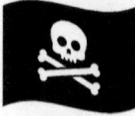

THE HIJACKER
Takes mentee's ideas, projects, or grants and **presents them as their own.**

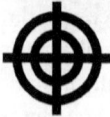

THE EXPLOITER
Offers only low-yield activities to mentee that will only advance the mentor's **own agenda.**

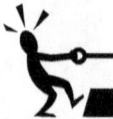

THE POSSESSOR
Prevents mentee from reaching out to others for guidance/collaboration, **seeing these as threats** to their expertise, influence, position, or rank.

PASSIVE

THE BOTTLENECK
Has zero time to mentor. Requires they sign off on mentee's work, **tying mentee to mentor's timeline.**

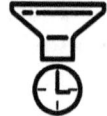

THE COUNTRY CLUBBER
Prioritizes agreeable relations and social standing. Avoids difficult conversations, often leading to **inadequate support** and **slowing mentee advancement.**

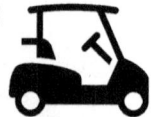

THE WORLD TRAVELER
Globetrots from keynote speeches to society leadership meetings, with **little time for mentee.** Can be a side effect of success.

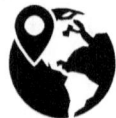

FIGURE 4.1 Six types of mentorship malpractice.

Active Mentorship Malpractice

There are three classic phenotypes of active mentorship malpractice, which all refer to the mentor taking an active role in diminishing the career and eroding the self-confidence of the mentee.

The Hijacker

These are the bullies who take the mentee's ideas, projects, or grants, and present or label them as their own. They do this for self-gain or self-preservation. Those who partake in these behaviors are often facing career challenges such as insufficient grant funding, limited academic output, lack of intellectual creativity, or promotion and tenure delays. In other words, these are often people in desperate situations.

Some mentees, while feeling uneasy about what has unfolded, might be complicit in this negative behavior. They feel valued that their work is good enough for the mentor to want to slap their name on it. The mentee, with little to no fight or power, might give up their rights to the product, feeling that the mentor's success will one day spill forward onto them.

Sadly, this spillover rarely happens. Rather, once a mentor commits this crime, they are likely to do it again. Before you know it, a mentee is sinking in academic quicksand. By the time they realize they have been cheated, the damage has been done, and it is hard, although not impossible, to recover.

The Exploiter

True learning occurs just beyond the edge of our comfort zone. This is often done by giving mentees stretch assignments that help them learn and grow. However, the exploiter does the exact opposite. They give the mentee low-yield activities that will not help them in their career. Rather, these activities help the mentor move their own agenda forward and keep their projects moving. Think of a PhD student washing glassware all day, a medical resident writing notes but not being allowed to present on rounds, or a junior investigator preparing their mentor's annual grant reports or protocol applications.

Exploiters tend to give their mentees the academic work they despise doing, such as taking minutes during research team meetings, submitting to IRB committees and responding to their queries, and setting up meetings that would be more appropriate for an administrative assistant to do. The mentors may justify it as a valuable learning experience, but without guidance and engagement, no learning or growth occurs. This nuance is critical: exploiters are all about getting the work done, not about getting it done in a way that helps a mentee grow.

Furthermore, exploiters may assign mentees to mentor students, supervise their projects, or manage some of the mentor's critical projects that are not within the interest or portfolio of the mentee. The exploiters see their mentees as free labor or managers and do nothing to cultivate the careers, let alone grow the knowledge and experience base of the mentee.

The Possessor

This mentor lacks self-confidence and dominates the mentee. They don't want the mentee talking to anyone else or seeking guidance from others, and they absolutely don't want to hear of collaborations. This tormentor mentor sees these opportunities as a threat to their expertise, influence, position, and rank.

Their jealousy and need for control often manifest in hurtful ways. We know of possessors who have prevented their mentees from attending high-profile conferences and meeting with key leaders in the field, or have discouraged meeting with peer mentors and colleagues to socialize their ideas.

Mentees who have been mentored by a possessor often have to isolate themselves from academic, social, or collegial gatherings or risk their mentor's wrath. This makes it difficult for anyone to see the signs and help them. Worse, they may even begin to identify with their mentor and promulgate this behavior.

Passive Mentorship Malpractice

Not all bad behavior by mentors is toxic or obvious. Rather, some is insidious and revolves around what the mentor *doesn't* do. Here, too, there are three archetypes.

The Bottleneck

These individuals are often too stretched to generate the interest or bandwidth to support a mentee. They like the "mentor" title but don't have a flicker of time or possess insanely poor time management skills, preventing them from being effective. They are so focused on their own goals that the mentee becomes an afterthought.

Their inability to offer any time to review goals, manuscripts, or presentations rapidly diminishes the mentee's productivity and feelings of accomplishment. This is incredibly problematic for mentees who are students or junior in their career and still have a long path ahead. To be clear, we have all been in situations where things get delayed or when life instances happen, getting in the way of timely feedback or responsiveness. The pathology with the Bottleneck is that delays are driven by lack of interest in the mentee.

This problem is quickly compounded when the Bottleneck also insists on signing off on the mentee's work, essentially assuring that the mentee's timeline is inextricably linked to theirs—or worse, on perpetual pause. Fast-forward several years, and a mentee with a Bottleneck mentor has little to show for their years of tutelage.

The Country Clubber

We all know this person. The one who never misses a holiday party, stops to talk with everyone in the hallway, and just wants to be liked by everyone. They avoid difficult conversations and simply want to be everyone's friend. This aversion to conflict is problematic as sometimes these difficult conversations are necessary. This is especially so when negotiating protected time for a mentee, battling for an authorship position, or ensuring adequate research support. Worse, not only do they avoid conflict; they often encourage the mentee to do the same even if that means they're losing out.

Country Clubbers see mentorship as a surrogate for social status. They use the number of mentees under their supposed tutelage as a bargaining chip to promote their social capital rather than focusing on ensuring their success. Mentees in these toxic relationships feel unsupported, smothered by always having to be the "nice guy/gal," and find it difficult to assert themselves—to the detriment of their career.

The World Traveler

Even during the COVID pandemic, when everyone was in lockdown, these mentors were busy virtually traveling the globe giving keynotes, actively participating in leadership roles in societies, or attending meetings. After travel restrictions subsided and pent-up demand for expertise swelled, these mentors found themselves spending more time away from the organization, leaving little time for mentees.

Ironically, the more successful the mentor becomes, the more susceptible they are to this type of mentorship malpractice. A lack of checking in with the mentee, even virtually, leaves mentees feeling adrift. The mentee feels mentorless from the lack of direction and interaction.

Consequences of Mentorship Malpractice

There are far-reaching ripple effects of mentorship malpractice, and they impact the mentee, the organization, and healthcare at large.

Personal Impact on Mentees

Those who have had a tormentor mentor and have been on the receiving end of mentorship malpractice might face burnout, loss of confidence, and significant career derailment.[4] Extreme cases can result in mental health consequences such as anxiety or depression.[11,12]

Organizational Impact

Positive mentoring is the best recruitment and retention tool out there. Studies have shown that those who are mentored are twice as likely to stay with an organization as those who are not.[13] It fosters loyalty, breeds trust, and secures competence. The opposite is also true. Poor mentorship results in increased turnover and loss of talented professionals.[12] Replacing talented employees is expensive, and there is a steep learning curve. Preventing a revolving door of healthcare workers due to poor mentorship should be a priority.

Trust and collaboration[14] are the bedrock of productive healthcare organizations. Toxic mentorship creates an erosion in the culture of trust and collaboration, leading to watercooler gossip, lack of engagement, and limited innovation due to the lack of collaboration.

Broader Consequences in Healthcare

When the mentees, who take care of patients and are at the forefront of innovative research, feel stepped on, put out, ignored, or diminished, there is a cascading negative impact on patient care and team performance.[15] This, we posit, may be one of the reasons for the mass exodus from healthcare resulting in significant doctor and nursing shortages. We are facing a problem of epic proportions, but we also have the tools to fix it.

How to Identify and Avoid Tormentor Mentors

Mentorship malpractice does not occur in a vacuum. For the dysfunctional relationship to occur, both the mentor and mentee, whether they know it or not, are willful participants. No pushback from the mentee gives the tormentor mentor the fuel they need to double down on their toxic ways.

Mentorship malpractice can be prevented and avoided through some key strategies, which we will discuss further in Chapter 10. Mentoring with mindfulness, as discussed in Chapter 15, will help place a mentor in the shoes of the mentee and avoid becoming a tormentor to them.

Creating a Culture That Prevents Mentorship Malpractice

Tormentor mentors should not be given free latitude to run rampant with their toxic traits. They *must* be reined in. Toxic behavior is contagious, like a virus, and research has shown it can spread dramatically.[16]

Healthcare organizations and their leaders must take this seriously. Telling people they need to mentor is not enough. Give them the proper resources and train them on how to be effective mentors and avoid mentorship malpractice. It doesn't matter how many mentees they've trained or how many people work in their lab. Lead workshops, give them books and articles, and provide access to resources. See the book's Appendix for a list of resources we recommend.

Summary

Mentorship malpractice is more than just a personal or professional setback—it is a systemic issue with far-reaching consequences for individuals, organizations, and the entire healthcare industry. The difference between a mentor and a tormentor can shape careers, influence workplace culture, and even impact patient outcomes in healthcare. Recognizing the warning signs of toxic mentorship, building a diverse mentoring team, and advocating for healthier mentorship dynamics are critical steps toward breaking the cycle of dysfunction. By fostering an environment of accountability, clear communication, and ethical guidance, we can shift mentorship from a source of stress and harm to one of growth, empowerment, and success. The responsibility lies with both mentors and mentees to create a culture where mentorship is not only effective but also transformative.

Take-Home Points

- Toxic mentorship environments are far too common, and they have a profound effect on a mentee's academic experience and career path. Unfortunately, negative behavior is rarely isolated—it's contagious.
- Mentorship malpractice can be either active or passive. Active malpractice seeks self-promotion and diminishes a mentee's accomplishments and confidence. Passive malpractice is characterized by inaction and squandering a mentee's talent and hard work as the mentor is "too busy" or doesn't follow through on their word.
- Toxic mentorship not only harms individual mentees but also has detrimental effects on the workplace culture and broader healthcare system. As trust erodes, collaboration declines, leading to increased turnover, and ultimately patient care suffers. Addressing mentorship malpractice is crucial to sustaining a positive, effective healthcare workforce.

5

Mentoring across Differences

Lata, a PhD candidate from India, was assigned to complete her dissertation under Steve, who had never worked with a student from Asia before. They would meet biweekly, and Steve would provide her with feedback on her experiments and data, which Lata vigorously scribbled into her notepad, nodding vehemently as she did so. The following week, she would modify her setup and do exactly as Steve said.

Steve was impressed at the follow-through but soon noticed that Lata was not bringing her ideas or creativity to the lab. He finally asked, "Lata, you do great work, but I don't see you trying to develop your own approach. You simply do as I say." Surprised, Lata replied, "That is my duty as your student—to follow your instructions." Steve had failed to appreciate the cultural norm—questioning a teacher could be considered poor form in Lata's country. Understanding this now, he said, "Lata, nothing I suggest is set in stone. I want you to ask me questions and propose different ideas at all of our meetings."

Why Mentoring across Differences Matters

When you think about mentoring, do you naturally picture someone similar to yourself? Many people do. Yet some of the most impactful mentoring relationships arise when individuals from different backgrounds come together to share knowledge, experiences, and perspectives.

Until recently, if you walked down the halls of most academic institutions, you'd notice that the portraits of most of the former leaders looked the same.[1] They were all generally Caucasian, male, and older—referred to on social media as the "dude wall."

As the workforce has changed, so too have senior roles. For the first time, we are consistently seeing women (who for years have made up about 50% of the medical school classes[2]) ascend to senior roles. Group photos of incoming classes of physicians, scientists, nurses, and every other sector of the healthcare workforce are now beginning to mirror the tapestry of the population that they serve. And so too do the pictures of those who lead labs, programs, divisions, and departments.

As a result, your mentors, and whom *you* mentor, are likely going to be different from yourself. But in the difference lies the strength. Mentoring across differences—whether in cultures, genders, ethnicities, political viewpoints, generations, or religions—can be one of the most powerful ways to grow as both a mentor and mentee. By engaging with those who think differently, we challenge our own perspectives, learn to embrace new approaches and ideas, foster innovation, and open doors for broader professional success. And mentees who were otherwise disenfranchised will learn what it takes to be successful, opening doors for themselves and their mentees to succeed. This chapter focuses on how to navigate these mentorship differences effectively, ensuring they remain grounded in respect, curiosity, and a genuine desire to support professional and personal growth.

Expanding Your Mentorship Mindset

Mentorship across differences starts with a perspective shift. Research consistently shows that people tend to naturally connect with those who look like them or have a similar background.[3,4] This is referred to as the similarity–attraction effect. While this approach might feel familiar and comfortable, it stagnates growth and innovation, as research has clearly shown that diverse teams are more effective, innovative, and profitable than homogeneous ones.[5-7] True and effective mentoring means we need to step outside our comfort zone and actively engage with perspectives and experiences that might be different from our own.

To do this effectively, there are three foundational steps to keep in mind:

1. **Recognize biases:** As Nobel Prize–winning psychologist Dr. Daniel Kahneman and Dr. Amos Tversky shared in their research, when making

judgments, we rely on mental shortcuts, which are influenced by our past experiences.[8] Consequently, we all have biases. Being aware that these exist and ensuring that we pause before making judgments are the first steps toward effective mentorship.[9]

2. **Lead with curiosity:** Don't assume, ask. Just because you, as the mentor, faced a challenge, doesn't mean your mentee faces the same challenges. Ask them what difficulties they are facing (Ruth's favorite question is, "What's keeping you up at night?"), and ask how you can best support them. Just like Steve finally asked Lata in our opening story, curiosity can allow for new understandings and new approaches to unfold.

3. **View mentorship as shared growth:** Mentorship is a symbiotic relationship. Both parties can gain new skills and perspectives from the other. While a mentor provides guidance, wisdom, resources, and encouragement based on past experiences, a mentee brings fresh ideas, angles, new technologies, and insights that can challenge conventional thinking. The most successful mentoring relationships evolve over time, shifting from a one-way knowledge transfer to a bidirectional exchange of ideas. Over time, the lines blur, and it may be difficult to recognize who is the mentor and who is the mentee. Vineet has been the beneficiary of this in almost all his mentoring relationships, and his extensive use of cloud-sharing solutions like Dropbox today are a result of such interactions.

Mentoring across Different Backgrounds

Ruth once mentored a group of physician leaders at a major hospital. One division chief proudly announced that he takes his mentees out for drinks and golf after work. The chief couldn't understand why the group who attended were all the same. Ruth inquired as to the makeup of the group. They were all mid-career and male. Ruth politely explained that not everyone likes golf, and likely fewer women than men own their own golf clubs. Secondly, after-work drinks are very challenging for those early in their career, as they run home to have dinner with their family, help their children with homework, and tuck them in for the night. While a nice gesture, the timing, location, and activity excluded certain groups. This division chief wasn't trying to exclude anyone; he was just not aware how to mentor people who are different from him. After all, almost all his colleagues in medical school and residency looked and behaved just like him and would have killed for an evening of drinks and golf!

The truth is that it's impossible to find a mentor or mentee who is identical to you in every way—same gender, cultural upbringing, socioeconomic background, political views, etc. Indeed, for mentoring to be effective, a foundation of trust, understanding, and mutual respect for differences is foundational.

As we tell many of our mentees, if you want to learn something new, go find someone who is different from you. See these differences as opportunities, not barriers. They can foster deeper connections and broaden perspectives. Seek to learn from prospective mentees by asking about their norms, work–life balance, and (if willing) their values. By approaching this conversation directly and embracing curiosity, cultural awareness, and an open mind, the relationship can be inclusive and meaningful for both parties, regardless of background.

While by no means an all–inclusive list, some of the most common differences in healthcare include:

1. **Cultural and ethnic differences:** Different cultures may have unique professional expectations, communication styles, and networking approaches. In some cultures, it's acceptable to be in close proximity when talking to someone, whereas in others, it's considered invasive and rude. Some cultures expect you to look the person in the eyes when talking to them, when in others, it's considered disrespectful. A good mentor takes the time to look for, ask about, and understand these nuances to ensure the effectiveness of the relationship.

2. **Religious differences:** Mentoring someone from a different religious background requires respect and awareness[10–12] of practices that may require them not to work or eat on certain days and prohibit certain foods. Every year, meetings are scheduled on the Jewish high holidays, conferences scheduled over Easter, and lunch receptions planned during daytime fasts of Ramadan. Lack of awareness of these norms may lead to a flurry of emails, apologies, and rapid changes when a quick Google search could have sufficed. Most human resources offices have these dates and norms identified for your organization. Mark them on your calendar, become aware of key religious observances of those under your tutelage, and avoid this unnecessary faux pas.

3. **Political viewpoints:** If ever there was a landmine, it is politics. People hold different political views, as is their right, and it is not the mentor or mentee's role to try to persuade the other in this area. Make this topic off limits and focus on professional growth and shared values rather than political alignment. If it does come up (as it often does), acknowledging

and respecting differences in ideology are important. We know of more than one mentoring relationship where politics became a divisive force and led to significant turbulence.

4. **Gender dynamics:** In her book, *In a Different Voice*, Dr. Carol Gilligan, explains that by the mere fact they are placed on competitive sports teams at an early age, men are conditioned to be competitive.[13] They understand the rules of the game and are playing to win. Women, on the other hand, are often raised to be collaborative, playing with one another, instead of against one another on the playground. As a result, they may not understand the rules of the game.

Especially if you are a male mentor who advises women, understand that women may face different hurdles than you, starting with the lack of familiarity[14] with the rules of the game.[15] Supporting them in standing up for their work and career and ensuring that they get and claim credit for work done should thus be a norm. Coach them to have conversations that may initially seem off-putting, such as asking for a raise or for a nicer office. The same applies for the approach to promotions, leadership roles, and other opportunities. Mentoring across gender[9] requires awareness, not fear.[16,17] Your job as a mentor is to help them grow and achieve their full potential. Open doors for them that they never knew existed, and then prepare them to shine once they get the role.[18]

Dr. Michelle Moniz and Sanjay have written[9] on how men can be effective allies for women by embracing the following three key behaviors: (1) being mindful of gender scripts, (2) embracing reciprocal learning, and (3) being the change we wish to see in the world by wielding social capital to advance policies that promote gender equity. Dr. Lona Mody, from the University of Michigan, wrote a paper[19] in a top-tier basic science journal on what female artists can teach scientists, in which she and her co-authors outlined the contributions of three female painters and what scientists can learn from each. The three artists are (1) Elisabeth Vigée Le Brun from France—know when to change course; (2) Mary Cassatt from the United States—go where the action is; and (3) Frida Kahlo from Mexico—our imperfections make us complete.

5. **Neurodiversity:** Mentoring neurodivergent individuals, such as those with autism, ADHD, dyslexia, or other cognitive differences, requires understanding and flexibility. Neurodivergent mentees may process information and communicate differently and problem-solve in unique ways. Effective mentors recognize and appreciate these differences, adapting their mentoring approaches to offer scaffolding to align with the mentee's strengths and processes to help with some of their challenges.[20] Having

a mentorship team with individuals who have skills and experience in mentoring similar individuals can be very helpful for all members.

Simple modifications such as having notes of the meeting with a summary action plan (there are AI tools that can do this for you), allowing extra processing time, and encouraging unconventional problem-solving techniques can make a real impact. By offering a mentoring environment where the mentee can thrive, you can unlock their full potential, while also learning new ways to approach challenges.

Ruth was mentoring someone with ADHD and processing challenges who was easily distracted. To be more effective in their meetings, they were always either in person or made use of video, in places where there were few distractions. Action plans with nudge reminders were sent after each meeting so that the mentee never missed deadlines. It gave them the tools to succeed.

6. **First-generation challenges:** Students who are the first in their family to attend college face many distinct challenges. They lack social capital, institutional knowledge, and professional networks. They are also unfamiliar with the hidden curriculum,[21] the unwritten rules and traditions that are passed down and known in certain circles—anything from the need to apply early for interviews to appropriate dress codes and social cues. Mentors are incredibly useful in acknowledging these barriers, offering tips on navigation, recommending career pathways that may be completely foreign to the mentee (as they've never even seen them before), and leveraging political capital by introducing mentees to those in the mentor's network.

First-generation students often have incredible drive and resilience, and mentors can help channel their energy properly. They can also clue the mentee in on unspoken workplace norms, connect them with resources, and offer encouragement when imposter syndrome strikes.

Practical Guidelines for Mentors

Recognizing and respecting differences are the first steps in effective mentorship. Next, you need to translate your awareness into actionable strategies that foster understanding and growth. Mentors should be intentional in their approach—adapting their style and ensuring that all mentees, irrespective of background, feel valued, included, and supported. We offer the following practical guidelines to help cultivate positive relationships. This is by no means an all-inclusive list, and we encourage you to add your own spin to it.

Take Stock of Your Mentoring Activities

The first step toward mentoring anyone is to be cognizant of providing equal opportunities to everyone. You might not even be aware that you are subconsciously leaving people out of receiving your guidance. Recall the story from earlier in the chapter about the mentor who took mentees to play golf. Or the story about Lata not offering feedback but following through as told. Of course, neither mentor meant to exclude anyone, but the selection of the activity and the after-work timing, as well as the failure to clarify expectations, meant certain groups were automatically excluded.

Mentoring, sponsoring, coaching, and building connections for people, regardless of their gender, how they look, what they believe, whom they voted for, and where they are from, are critical. Be mindful of your own practice and personal biases (again, we all have them) and try to distribute your time, energy, and accolades as equitably as possible, keeping in mind what each mentee needs and how they learn best. (We will discuss that later in the chapter.)

It's also important to know that some individuals may not seek out mentorship as aggressively as others. Studies have shown that women are less likely to request mentorship or sponsorship than their male counterparts.[22,23] In some cultures, asking for help is seen as a sign of weakness. It is up to the mentor to keep a watchful eye for undiscovered talent. If you don't have a mentee table, create one and color-code individuals for certain aspects (e.g., colors for gender, scientific area of focus, country of origin, etc.). A visual such as this (akin to a "heat map") can help you spot gaps or "lack of a rainbow" when it comes to your mentees!

Adapt Your Mentorship Styles

Not everyone takes in and processes information in the same way. We're not talking about auditory versus tactile learners, which has been debunked.[24] Consider the Kolb Learning Style,[25] which underscores the idea that some people take in information by reading or listening, but might process things by reflecting privately or by talking them out. The point is that a one-size-fits-all model won't work. Some mentees want to talk through their challenge until they get to their aha moment with the mentor's guidance. Others like to brainstorm independently and may email you their ideas for feedback. Both are valid.

Dr. Ellie Drago-Severson's work on adult development[26] reminds us that, while some mentees might need their mentors' validation, others are looking for guidance. Some might see your feedback as criticism, while others will see it as data points that they will use to make their own independent decisions. Again, both are correct options, which reminds us that you should not mentor each mentee the same way. Rather, asking them about how they approach key issues such as feedback, learning, and strategic advice can help clarify this relationship and avoid harm.

Be aware of how your mentee takes in and processes information (it's okay to ask them), and adapt your mentoring style accordingly.

Create Safe Conversations

At the core of a mentoring relationship is trust. The mentee has to feel that they can approach their mentor without the feeling of judgment or fear of criticism—what Harvard Business School professor Dr. Amy Edmondson refers to as psychological safety.[27]

To create a safe space so that you can have the most productive mentoring conversations, consider the following:

- **Encourage open-ended questions that invite honest discussions:** Questions that have yes/no answers can abruptly cut off conversations and make them feel more like an interrogation. Instead, consider questions that start with "how," "what," or "why."

- **Actively listen without interrupting or making assumptions:** Listen to both what is said and what is omitted. Give them the time and space to respond—and expect them to have a reaction so that this is normalized as part of the discussion.

- **Refrain from judgment and validate your mentee's experiences:** Just because it didn't happen to you doesn't mean it can't happen to others.

- **Confidentiality is non-negotiable:** Your mentee needs to believe that anything they tell you will not be shared without their permission. Especially when it comes to cultural norms or behaviors (e.g., prayers at fixed hours) that may make the mentee uncomfortable if known to a broader audience.

- **Watch for non-verbal cues—body language can tell a lot:** Be on the lookout for signals from your mentee—perhaps they won't look you in the eye or try to make themselves small by hunching over and crossing their legs. Conversely, as a mentor, you should always make sure that the way you hold yourself conveys openness and support, such as trying to avoid crossing your arms or looking at your computer or phone while your mentee is talking to you. If you see something that makes you think the discussion is no longer comfortable, pause and ask about it. It may help save many a heartache later!

- **Phrase feedback as an opportunity for growth, not critique:** Athletes crave feedback[28] as they know that any tip could mean the difference between getting a medal and staying off the podium. Express feedback as a way to make them better, not to critique past performance.

Avoid Exclusive Networking

Make sure all of your mentees, regardless of background, have access to professional opportunities, such as conferences, informal gatherings, and valuable professional events. Avoid the tendency to only invite your favorite, those who always seem to be available, or those with whom you are the most comfortable. In fact, when organizing social events, invite them all so they can engage with you and with one another and enrich the group.

Many professional connections happen in informal settings such as the bar or golf course. Be mindful that these types of activities might exclude certain mentees due to their cultural, financial, or parental responsibilities. Consider times and places that are more inclusive. And if you don't know what one may be? Ask!

Introduce your mentees to key professional contacts and be sure to prepare them[29] so they know how to behave and make the most of these professional connections. After all, this is your social and political capital, and you want them to honor and respect that. Teach them how to start these conversations. (Ruth has a list on her website of some great conversation starters: ruthgotian.com/conversation.) Recognize that these connections can be especially useful for those who may not have regular access to these types of networks.

Practical Guidelines for Mentees

Build a Diverse Mentoring Team

While having a single mentor is certainly helpful, it is also limiting. As previously discussed, a mentoring team,[20] built with people who are senior to you, junior to you, and peers, is pivotal for diversity of thoughts and perspectives. Mix in people from within and outside your industry to really get a 360-degree view of how things could be done. If everyone on your mentoring team looks like you and has a similar background, you will be in an echo chamber, and the ideas and guidance you receive will be severely hampered.

Handle Difficult Conversations

Mentorship is a relationship, and in every relationship, problems will inevitably bubble up. The best mentors see these and call them out. Disagreements can be productive if handled appropriately.[28] They are not meant to critique; rather, they can steer you toward a new and bigger pathway. These conversations are opportunities for enhancement. Approach these conversations with respect and focus on the shared goals. It's less about what you did wrong, and more about how to do things right, in a bigger, better, more impactful way.

Overcoming Self-Doubt and Imposter Syndrome

No, the admissions committee did not make a mistake, and no one is withdrawing any offers. When times get tough, we often default to thinking we can't hack it. When something good happens, we default to thinking it was random luck, and we'll be seen as a fraud. That's imposter syndrome and is common in about 70% of people, including actor Tom Hanks, Supreme Court Justice Sonya Sotamayor, literary giant JK Rowling, and former first lady Michelle Obama. If you are feeling like an imposter, you're in good company.

When this happens, talk to your mentor, and review your achievements. Before long, you will notice that you earned your accolade, and the imposter syndrome should serve as a source of strength and pride, not anxiety.[30]

Leveraging Peer Networks

While support often comes from senior mentors, it is often your peers who offer the greatest empathy and so are an integral part of the mentoring team. They are going through the same or very similar work-related pressures and understand what you are feeling. They can become powerful listeners and share what worked, or didn't, for them.

If you mixed up your mornings and nights after being on call, or you always feel you haven't read and studied enough before a case, your peers were likely feeling similar stresses in the not so distant past. Lean on them and allow them to lean on you.

By broadening our mentoring networking beyond those who mirror our own looks and experiences, we create strong, more inclusive, and professional environments that benefit the individual and our organizations.

Summary

Mentoring across differences matters because it opens doors for innovation and broader professional success. Historically, leadership and mentor roles have lacked diversity. However, recent shifts show diverse, inclusive leadership in healthcare, which mirrors the diverse population that healthcare providers serve, though opportunities to be mentored may still not be equally available to those of different genders, race, or cultural background.[31]

Mentors should recognize their biases, lead with curiosity, and appreciate differences as strengths, offering guidance without judgment. It's important for them to ensure inclusivity by adapting mentorship styles and fostering safe conversations. For mentees, building a diverse mentoring team is crucial for understanding varied perspectives.

Engaging with mentors and mentees from different backgrounds enriches both parties, enhancing growth through shared experiences and challenges. Mentors should be intentional in their approach, adapting their mentoring style to ensure all mentees, regardless of background, feel valued, included, and supported.

Take-Home Points

- By engaging with those who have different viewpoints, we challenge our own perspectives and welcome new approaches and ideas, fostering innovation and creating opportunities for broader professional success.
- A foundation of trust, understanding, and mutual respect for differences is foundational. Ensure your mentorship conversations are a safe place for mentees to learn, pitch new ideas, and grow.
- Mentoring, sponsoring, coaching, and building connections for people, regardless of their gender, how they look, what they believe, who they voted for, and where they are from, are critical. Do you give equal opportunities to everyone?

6

Mentoring in a Virtual Era

Gone may be the days of a formal mentoring meeting occurring at a given time or place. The way we mentor others has had a complete overhaul—something that was done out of sheer necessity. While in-person mentoring has long been the gold standard in healthcare, the shift to hybrid and remote work, as well as work hour rules, have forced the entire healthcare industry to reimagine how we connect, guide, and develop the next generation of healthcare workers. But in this reorganization is also an opportunity to expand mentorship beyond geographic barriers and traditional hierarchies.

Traditionally, in healthcare, mentoring could be recognized for having three components:

1. **Apprenticeship model:** Working one-on-one under the guidance of a senior healthcare worker in your field has been a hallmark of mentoring. This more senior incumbent would provide direct observation of your work, hands-on practice, and real-time feedback. Think of a resident or fellow with a surgeon in the operating room. The fellow performs a maneuver during the procedure, the surgeon watches and gives feedback in real time so that the fellow can immediately make adjustments.

2. **Hierarchical relationships:** Typically, a senior physician, researcher, or colleague would mentor someone more junior. These types of mentoring relationships occur every day on rounds and in class teachings, as well as at informal teaching moments.

3. **Physical proximity:** Being located close to your mentor's office allows for spontaneous learning opportunities, ranging from case discussions to ethical considerations in real time. In fact, many career development awardees often highlight this close physical proximity in their grant

DOI: 10.1201/9781003611233-7

applications, recognizing it as a critical component of their training environment.

In 2003, the Accreditation Council for Graduate Medical Education (ACGME) passed the work hour rules,[1] limiting, for the first time, the number of work hours for physicians in training. This led to pre- and post-call days off as well as other changes to the training of residents and fellows. The COVID-19 pandemic emergence in 2020 escalated, nearly overnight, the use of remote and hybrid work at scale. It also made us rethink how we can and may mentor going forward.

Tech-Enabled Mentorship

While there are still some facets of the apprenticeship model in certain areas of healthcare, the hierarchical relationships and need for physical proximity have become less common. Becoming comfortable with virtual communication and collaboration tools such as Zoom, Teams, Slack, Loom, and texting has allowed mentors and mentees to find each other[2] and work together beyond the walls of their organization, state, and even country. The only thing that seems to stop someone now is the lack of a reliable internet connection.

Artificial intelligence (AI) is the new tool that has created a paradigm shift in mentoring.[3] Beyond using it as a tool to match mentors and mentees, it can create learning plans and skill recommendations and track progress. It is great for providing transcripts, action items lists, and nudges for things you promised to do. No need to worry who will take notes and keep track of action items. Certainly, AI can do that well. And, increasingly, tools like Microsoft Copilot provide feedback on your day, activities, meetings, and work output. These tools are thus here to stay.

Artificial intelligence can help connect people across platforms and create transcripts of meetings, notes, and even project outlines and calendars. However, machines cannot replace empathy and human connection, the foundations of unshakable mentoring relationships. Simply put, AI is a technical but not social tool. By all means, however, leverage technology to expand your mentorship's reach, connect with diverse mentees across the globe, and form mentoring teams that cross time zones and borders. Use the progress tools to identify and celebrate achievements, and, of course, utilize AI's many features to save you time and energy on administrative burdens.

Asynchronous versus Synchronous Mentorship

Varying call and meeting schedules mean mentors and mentees may not be available at the same time or place. This brings up a great point—not all mentoring needs to occur in tandem. Whether in person or virtually, there are many opportunities to engage in synchronous (meaning live) meetings, case discussions, Grand Rounds, and teaching rounds. The ability to connect with tools such as Zoom allows you to *be* there, without actually being present in the same room.

Technology has allowed for the opportunity to engage in mentorship in an asynchronous format. Watching recorded lectures, providing digital feedback, notes on manuscript or grant proposals, emails, and text messages are all acceptable ways of communicating and mentoring asynchronously.

Breaking Down Barriers

Ruth, who lives in the United States, was working on a manuscript with someone who lived in New Zealand. Getting the time zones aligned for a Zoom meeting was a serious challenge, so after an initial call, they reverted to email. Because of the time difference, they were essentially working consistently in 24-hour shifts. Ruth would work on the manuscript and email it to her co-author in New Zealand. When Ruth was leaving for the day, her colleague in New Zealand was starting hers. By the time Ruth returned in the morning, there were edits to review. The enormous time zone difference worked to their advantage, allowing them to finish the project in less time.

There might be times when you need someone with a certain skillset, experience, or network, and they might be in another organization or country. In the "old days" that person may not have been someone you could consider as a mentor. Virtual mentoring now removes those barriers and allows you to communicate with someone down the hall or across the globe with ease. This is especially useful as it provides greater flexibility and, in some cases, greater efficiency.

Challenges of Virtual Mentorship in Healthcare

While virtual mentorship offers accessibility and flexibility, it also has some challenges, especially in healthcare, where the learning is at times necessarily hands-on, and the feedback and problem solving are best done in real time. Traditional mentoring thrives on spontaneous interactions in the operating room, discussions in the team room, brief hallway chats, and even body language cues. In a virtual setting, these impromptu opportunities often vanish, requiring mentoring to be more intentional.

Beyond the physical space, there are also logistical and technological challenges. Not every healthcare professional has the same level of digital fluency, and, let's face it, dead zones for phone calls and internet connections are a reality. Furthermore, trust, the foundation of a mentoring relationship, takes longer to build when interactions are confined to the screen. If we're not careful, the virtual mentoring can feel transactional instead of transformational. It is also hard to read cultural or emotional cues in virtual settings—which is why we always recommend "camera on" if you are going to engage in virtual sessions.

Best Practices for Effective Virtual Mentorship

Great mentorship is less about the platform and more about the connection. In a technology-fueled virtual setting, how that connection is established and maintained is critical. As impromptu chats are replaced with scheduled communication, you want to ensure that the mentoring does not become transactional. For virtual mentoring to be effective, you need to be strategic. Choose the right tools, set clear expectations, create engaging conversations, and foster a true connection despite the digital divide. When done correctly, virtual mentoring can be just as effective as in-person mentoring—perhaps more so, as it removes barriers such as time constraints, accessibility, and geography. While there are endless fancy tools out there, we find that the tried-and-true communication tools that are commonly used lower the barrier to entry and, frankly, will get used. We provide a list of the most commonly used tools in effective mentoring.

Choosing the Right Technology

You wouldn't use IV fluids to treat heart failure. The same is true when selecting technology for your mentoring conversations and tracking your work. More is not better. New is not necessarily better either. Rather, a nuanced approach is often needed. While technology is always changing, we wanted to offer tools that we use regularly at the time of writing this book.

Video Calls

Zoom and Microsoft Teams dominate the market and work well for discussions and group conversations. We also routinely use these platforms to share documents that you can both see and edit during the call. There is also the availability of an AI tool such as Otter.ai or Fathom to provide a transcript and action points resulting from the discussion, allowing you to focus squarely on the person and the work. However, note that some hospital systems will turn off this AI feature, due to HIPAA. If that is the case, the traditional video platforms will offer a basic transcription of the meeting, if you turn on that feature. Importantly, when you choose video, the cameras must be on.

Messaging Apps

Slack, WhatsApp, and Signal are great for quick check-ins, ongoing short form communication, and real-time problem solving. We like the WhatsApp group messaging feature as well and (in fact) used it as we were planning the various pieces of this book! Group messaging is also a great way to connect mentorship teams that may be separated across time and space. Messaging apps are especially helpful during air travel, as more and more flights offer Wi-Fi. You can solve a problem before you land, with a quick series of texts. Sanjay and Vineet have often had entire mentoring sessions on text when they've been in different corners of the world or in the air!

Collaboration Platforms

It is not uncommon for mentors and mentees to write papers or apply for grants together. Whether tracking goals, sharing documents, or keeping tabs on progress, Google Drive, DropBox, Microsoft One Drive, SharePoint, Box, and Trello are all popular tools. Choose a platform that works well for both of you (and one that you can master so as to train future mentees).

Avoid Tech Overload and Zoom Fatigue

Too much of anything is depleting. No one can be on Zoom all day or at their desk jumping from one technological tool to another. To avoid tech overload and Zoom fatigue, rotate between synchronous tools such as Zoom and asynchronous options such as email. Don't be shy about establishing some tech boundaries to prevent burnout. Consider limiting the number of Zoom calls you can have per day or what hours you prefer to schedule them. And keep them on the leaner side in terms of time. It's hard to see yourself (although you can hide the self-view) and keep talking to a screen for prolonged periods of time!

Structuring Virtual Mentorship Meetings

Lack of structure for mentoring meetings will lead to problems regardless of whether the meeting is in person or virtual. However, virtual meetings are especially dependent on having a robust structure. Our experience is that if you don't have some structure to the mentoring meetings, then you wind up wasting time and discussing little of consequence. Whether in person or virtual, random and unstructured meetings rarely work out well. To prevent this from occurring, consider putting these safeguards in place. (We also discuss this in more detail in Chapter 7.)

Setting a Clear Agenda

It's the mentee's responsibility to come to any mentoring meeting with a clear idea of the topic(s) they wish to discuss. Perhaps it is a challenge or an opportunity they are considering. Mentioning it upfront will ensure the entire time is not spent discussing a new movie that just came out or a recent vacation destination. It is best for the mentee to send the agenda (see Chapter 1 for a sample agenda) or at least the topics of discussion, in advance. The more complex and challenging the issue or the more pre-reading that is needed, the more time a mentor will need. Ask for your mentee to send materials ahead of meetings to allow time to reflect, posit solutions, and engage key stakeholders, including people in your network who might be useful to meet this goal or solve the challenge. If the agenda asks for feedback on work products, make sure there's enough time for and access to any pre-reads so that you can come prepared to the meeting.

Meet at Recurring Times

If a mentee knows they are meeting monthly or biweekly, it allows them to prepare topics for discussions and material to be reviewed. These in-depth meetings allow for long-term goal setting and deep analysis, which takes preparation. Having a date on the calendar lets the mentee know when they need to have things prepared. Quick questions can be reserved for between the formal meetings.

Active Listening and Communication Techniques

Just because the mentee is talking, doesn't mean the mentor is listening, and vice versa. You have precious time to be together and strategize. For every minute to count, you need to have some communication strategies and know what to avoid. Multitasking is even more of a potential problem with virtual meetings—it takes discipline by both parties to avoid this.

Reflective Listening and Asking the Right Questions

When one person finishes speaking, summarize what you heard to ensure understanding and agreement. Try saying, "What I am hearing you say is . . . ."

To get the mentee to think deeply and perhaps come up with the solution on their own, consider asking them open-ended questions (those that can't be answered with a yes/no response). If they are stuck in their thinking, ask them questions such as, "I wonder what would happen if . . . ."

Establish Virtual Ground Rules

Setting clear guidelines and understanding proper Zoom etiquette can help make your meetings run more smoothly by avoiding awkward pauses and interruptions. Early in your mentorship, discuss and determine which rules to implement. For instance, using Zoom's "reactions" feature to raise your hand before speaking, appointing a meeting moderator for group sessions, or ensuring meeting codes so you don't get "Zoom bombed" can all be effective ground rules for virtual communication.

Additionally, you might consider setting expectations for camera usage, muting microphones when not speaking, and (for a group) designating specific times for questions to maintain a focused and efficient meeting flow. By laying this groundwork, you create a more professional and productive virtual work environment.

Digital Distractions

We are all at fault. Our devices have an allure that's addicting. But multitasking, such as checking your email or scrolling on social media, during virtual mentorship calls minimizes engagement and is simply rude. If you haven't yet figured it out, the person you are talking to can always tell if you are multitasking. (Your eyes give it away!) You are looking away and not fully engaged. It's impossible to hide your distraction. When you're mentoring on Zoom, turn on your camera, put on your microphone (assuming you are in a quiet location), and focus purely on the meeting.

Consider putting your devices on "do not disturb" so they don't constantly ring and ping. Perhaps put a similar "do not disturb" sign on your door when you're in meetings so that people don't pop in with a "quick question."

Note taking, while necessary, can also reduce the focus. As discussed earlier in the chapter, if notes are a must, consider using an AI tool to take notes and come up with the action items and list the responsible person for each task.

Fostering Personal Connection in a Digital Space

During the COVID pandemic, people got *very* creative in how they met up—virtual coffees, dinners, painting parties, story times, and so much more. The same can be done with mentoring. Consider having virtual coffee chats, virtual drop-in office hours, or even designated times to chat about non-work-related matters to build rapport. Encourage your mentees to share personal stories and career aspirations, beyond their immediate goals. Lead by example by being vulnerable and sharing what you are working on. Perhaps you are training for a marathon, learning a new language, or learning how to meditate. Use storytelling (of real stories) and shared experiences to build connection and trust. Mentees often don't think of their mentors as human—providing that personal story of a struggle often goes a long way.

Build Psychological Safety

For mentorship to work, the mentee has to feel comfortable with their mentor. They should never feel like they are being judged and should be able to open up and be vulnerable. This ability to share concerns without fear of retribution is what Harvard Business School's Dr. Amy Edmondson refers to as *psychological safety*.[4] Validate their feelings, and show you are here to help, not judge.

Hybrid Mentorship Models: Merging the Best of Both Worlds

Late night calls, just before or after Grand Rounds, and those "constructive collisions" that occur when you run into people in the hallways or between clinic patients are often where mentoring relationships take root. Having a mentor who really "gets" you, pushes you to grow, and encourages you is at the heart of a thriving mentoring relationship. It is based on personal connection. Being able to observe and interact in real time fosters a relationship that is difficult, although not impossible, to replicate through a screen.

But always being there is simply not feasible. Mentoring doesn't have to be either/or when it comes to in-person versus virtual. You can, and should, do both—a hybrid solution is a powerful one.

A hybrid mentoring model allows the mentor and mentee to leverage the convenience and accessibility of virtual meetings while also benefiting from the in-person, more intimate, and nuanced conversation. If your mentor is not in the same organization as you, planning an in-person coffee or meal at an annual conference is a perfect opportunity to get together and ideate. Hybrid mentorship is not a compromise; it's a strategic advantage that allows for structure, impactful mentoring that circumvents some of the constraints of geography or schedules.

How Hybrid Mentorship Works: Combining In-Person and Virtual Touchpoints

With hybrid mentoring, keep three ideas in mind to make sure things don't get lost and that time together is efficient.

1. **Structured approach:** Set a regular cadence for virtual check-ins and periodic in-person meetings. Will you meet biweekly virtually and once a quarter in person, perhaps at a regional or national symposium you are both attending or at a common location if it's midway?
2. **Maximize each format:** Consider what types of activities you will do in person versus virtually. Perhaps *virtual sessions* will be for regular updates, structured learning, and discussion of projects and papers. Then *in-person meetings* can be for skill building, hands-on training, and deeper relationship building.
3. **Leverage technology to bridge the gap:** Productivity tools, such as shared dashboards, storage drives, and the messaging apps we discussed earlier, are all fantastic for maintaining continuity and transparency.

Measuring Success in Virtual Mentorship

Success takes time—it's like marinating food on a low flame. But eventually it happens, and it's glorious. A paper is published, a promotion secured, or confidence is built. The challenge is that it is not instant and is sometimes difficult to measure. And if you are virtual, you may not see the progress as clearly as you may in person.

That's why tracking progress is essential. Without proper metrics, virtual mentoring might be well-intentioned but lack depth. Both mentors and mentees need clear goals and feedback loops to ensure they are progressing on their agreed-upon agendas. But you can't just tick a box on a to-do list. You also need to engage, make introductions, and have a listening ear.

Tracking Progress and Setting Goals

Use SMART goals to guide your mentorship. SMART goals—specific, measurable, achievable, relevant, and time-bound—are a tried-and-true method for meeting goals. They provide a structured approach to goal attainment by turning abstract aspirations into clear, actionable objectives.

Instead of setting a vague goal, such as "improve leadership skills," a mentee in healthcare might use the SMART approach and say, "Lead three patient case discussions in the next six months and receive feedback from peers and supervisors." This specificity gives both mentor and mentee a clear objective, making progress easier to track. By setting milestones, regularly assessing achievements, and adjusting as needed, SMART goals keep virtual mentorship focused, intentional, and results driven. See Table 6.1 for an example of how SMART goals are used for mentoring in healthcare.

TABLE 6.1 Applying SMART Goals in Healthcare Mentoring

Component	Description	Example
Specific	Clearly defined	*Medical Resident*: Perform 5 supervised laparoscopic procedures during rotation
Measurable	Has criteria to track against	*Nurse Practitioner*: Collect feedback on their communication skills from 10 patients
Achievable	Realistic, given skills and resources	*Junior Researcher*: Co-author one research paper over the next year
Relevant	Aligns with career growth and professional responsibilities	*Physician*: Teach telemedicine protocols to prepare mentee to provide virtual care
Time-Bound	Has clear deadline to ensure accountability	*Hospital Administrator*: Develop a new staff mentorship program within 6 months

Feedback and Evaluations

A mentee needs to know how they are doing, and they need to understand that feedback is a tool for growth, not criticism.[5] When giving feedback, consider offering what leadership coach Dr. Marshall Goldsmith calls *feedforward*. Instead of focusing on the past, which cannot change, focus on the future. What ideas do you have to make things better, bigger, or more impactful? Given what has happened, what will we do differently as we look ahead if/when that same issue arises? This type of action-oriented feedback is much more powerful than an "I wish you had done xxxx . . . ." response.

Don't wait for the end of the year to give feedback. Give it in real time, and help the mentee reflect and consider how to improve things. After virtual meetings, consider promptly sending a follow-up email, summarizing key points, and including actionable next steps. Some personal feedback may be better suited for in-person meetings—aim to address these at your next face-to-face meeting, when able.

Qualitative Metrics

Engagement surveys, satisfaction reports, and qualitative evaluations of communication and work can all be used to help the mentee improve. Thankfully, these can easily be done in a virtual context. Choose an evaluation tool that suits both you and your mentee, and establish a regular schedule, such as annually or quarterly, to conduct these evaluations. When reviewing the results, focus on identifying overarching themes, rather than fixating on individual comments.

In Chapter 14, you will find a variety of methods for assessing the effectiveness of mentorship meetings, including approaches for group mentorship evaluations. A triangulated evaluation approach—which combines quantitative data, qualitative insights, and other relevant information—offers the most comprehensive and accurate measurement of your mentorship meetings and relationships.

Future of Virtual Mentorship in Healthcare

The way we learn, lead, treat others, and mentor in healthcare is evolving rapidly. With the advancement of AI, telehealth, and automation, everything as we know it is changing. While traditional in-person mentoring has been at the cornerstone of healthcare, virtual and hybrid mentorship have emerged as viable solutions to deal with on-call schedules, geographical limitations, and other such barriers. Yet, with all the talk of artificial intelligence and virtual work, human connection and empathy remain undisputed hallmarks of strong mentoring relationships.

Summary

Virtual communication and collaboration tools have forever left their mark on the development of mentorship. Geographical distance and hierarchy are no longer limiting factors, given the growing comfort with technology like Zoom, Teams, and Slack. Even barriers such as time zones are minimizing, as asynchronous collaborations become more common. However, virtual mentorship is not without its challenges. Mentoring effectively in a virtual format requires intentional structuring, using appropriate tools, establishing clear expectations, and fostering authentic connections. Hybrid mentorship models, however, can create a strategic advantage by blending the benefits of virtual sessions and occasional in-person meetings.

Whether virtual or hybrid, success in mentorship depends on structure, fostering connection, setting specific, measurable goals, and embracing continuous feedback. Despite the reality of an ever-evolving virtual environment, human connection remains at the core of mentorship.

Take-Home Points

- Mentorship has been transformed by the shift to virtual and hybrid work. Tools like Zoom remove the geographical and hierarchical barriers, and opportunities to mentor—or be mentored by—individuals outside your area are greater than ever. Consider whether an asynchronous workflow might work well for you and your mentee to accomplish a goal.
- Virtual mentoring presents its own set of challenges. Personal connection, including spontaneous touchpoints and live feedback, are often lacking, making it harder to establish trust. Instead, be proactive—structure virtual meetings well. Set a regular schedule, choose appropriate technology, establish ground rules, protect your time together, and listen well. Follow up meetings with an email summarizing the next steps.
- Hybrid mentorship models combine the best of both worlds, offering the advantages of scheduled virtual sessions for regular updates and discussion on projects and papers, while in-person meetings can provide deeper relationship building and time for personal feedback.

II

Becoming a Standout Mentee

7

The Mentee's Quick-Start Guide

The first meeting David (not his real name) had with his mentor was a mess. He was all over the place. He started off talking about his project, then quickly veered toward how difficult his week on hospital duty was and how exhausted he felt. Plus, his wife's birthday was coming up, and he hadn't even begun to plan what they were going to do. By the time the mentoring session was over, the mentor felt as exhausted and overwhelmed as David.

A common aphorism, derived from Buddhism, is, "When the student is ready, the teacher will appear." The teacher, in this case the mentor, is always ready with guidance, perspective, and experience, but until the mentee is ready, they will likely fall on deaf ears.

If the mentee wants the mentor's time and guidance and access to their network, they need to show that they are committed and worthy of such focused attention. They ideally need to come prepared for the meetings with a specific challenge or opportunity they'd like to discuss. They should demonstrate to the mentor through both words and actions that they've already invested time into the problem and have gotten as far as they can on their own. This allows for the discussion to build on a solid foundation rather than be a rambling narrative of disconnected thoughts and ideas.

Some may assume that the mentor bears the primary responsibility in a mentoring relationship, but this is not entirely accurate. Just as effective leadership stems from strong followership,[1] a successful mentor–mentee relationship thrives on an engaged, productive, and trustworthy mentee. In fact, the mentee is the one who drives the relationship forward and "manages up" when it comes to the mentor.

DOI: 10.1201/9781003611233-9

A mentor is not there to fix your life. Many mentees make a critical error by failing to recognize that they should at least try to bring their "A-game" to the mentoring relationship. They need to be all-in, or it doesn't work effectively. If the mentee's effort is half-baked, it will appear as if they don't care about their career or value the time of their mentor. And if the mentee doesn't care, why should the mentor? Without the mentee's best effort, the relationship will likely disintegrate and lead to career difficulties and even personal strife. A once promising career can ultimately be derailed as a result. Additionally, mentees risk missing a crucial opportunity for growth and insight—impacting not only their career but also those of their mentors and the advancement of the field.

Much of the academic literature on mentorship focuses on ideal mentor behaviors.[2-5] Our view is that the mentee's role in the relationship is often overlooked and undersubscribed. As the mentoring relationship is asymmetrical, mentees naturally have more to lose than their mentors if the mentoring relationship sours. Thus it behooves them to develop a blueprint by which they can plan, take action, and evaluate their growth.[6] With this in mind, here are some steps to ensure a mentee can develop a rewarding relationship.

Choose Your Mentor Wisely

Not every offer is worth accepting. Just as a mentor should select the right mentee, you should also be intentional when picking a potential mentor. As discussed in Chapter 4, selecting the wrong mentor could derail your career and take a toll on your confidence and mental health. Finding the right fit in a mentor[7] is especially important for your "traditional mentor," while the criteria for coaches, sponsors, and connectors can be more flexible.

What are the signs that a mentor is a good fit?[8] Before committing to a mentor, ask yourself the 12 questions laid out in Figure 7.1.

If you are not encouraged by the responses to these questions, you should carefully consider whether this mentor is really the best fit for you. It's better to take your time and find the right mentors[9] than to force an outcome from a mismatched relationship. Those rarely work out, so invest the time in your due diligence. Just be mindful that you don't turn down every single potential mentor because they're not a perfect fit. No one is perfect. But who will boost you and your career? A critical predictor is their track record: how well they have done for others.

WHAT ARE THE SIGNS THAT A MENTOR IS A GOOD FIT?

Before committing to a mentor, ask yourself these questions:

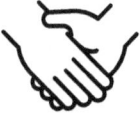

Is this a person I look up to, respect, and want to emulate?

Do their skills, priorities, and expertise align with my goals?

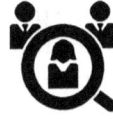

Does this person have a good track record mentoring others?

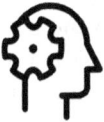

Do they challenge me to think critically and push me to grow?

Does the way they communicate work for me?

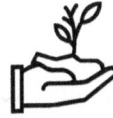

Are they willing and able to invest time and effort into my development?

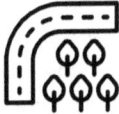

Do they want to pick my path, or help me find my own?

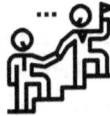

Can they provide robust mentorship on leadership, networking, etc.?

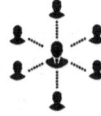

Are they willing and able to help me form and be part of my mentorship team?

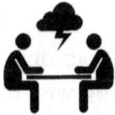

Is the way they handle challenges also the way that I want to work?

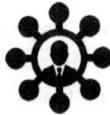

Are they respected, connected, & open to helping me network?

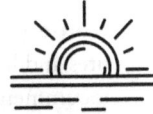

Does their feedback help me grow, or is it just flattery?

FIGURE 7.1 Twelve signs that a mentor is a good fit.

Be Mindful of Your Mentor's Time—Starting Now

If you've chosen an exceptional mentor, there's a good chance that their plate runneth over. A good rule of thumb is that your mentor is often far busier than you might think. Most great mentors are highly accomplished in their field. They are often juggling multiple roles and responsibilities. And they have the same 24 hours in the day as the rest of us. The best mentors make it look easy, but it most certainly is not. They are highly organized, efficient, and disciplined with their time to make it all work.

Despite their packed schedules, great mentors are authentically enthusiastic about investing their time into mentoring rising stars. This gives them great joy and is part of the journey of academia that makes careers impact-ful. However, being willing to mentor you doesn't mean they have the bandwidth or patience to hold your hand as you navigate every hiccup and hurdle. Your mentor's time is their most precious resource: You must use it wisely and productively. Best to first try and solve the problem on your own and propose a few solutions, rather than to run to the mentor and dump it on their plate half-baked. Making the effort shows that you took the initial steps, allows for mentors to correct or inform your thinking, and makes you more independent the next time you face the same challenge.

How can you make the most of every moment with your mentor?

1. **Schedule regular meetings on their calendar:** Determine a cadence for the meetings by asking them what makes the most sense. Ask them who coordinates their calendar and set up these meetings to avoid ex-changing endless emails. When the meetings are fixed, say the first and third Mondays of every month, other meetings get scheduled around that, as fixed meetings become a priority. Agree with your mentor to a regular rotation of meetings—and stick to it.

2. **Come prepared:** As time is precious, you need to maximize the min-utes and hours spent with your mentor. Regardless of your time slot, we recommend having no more than two to four topics you wish to discuss with your mentor as most topics will take 10–15 minutes to discuss. (We'll discuss some ideal topics and themes later in this chapter.) A pro-posed agenda for the meeting with relevant background information on the topics you wish to discuss is critical. See Chapter 1 for what a sample agenda could look like. This helps prepare your mentor for the meeting while ensuring you prioritize what's most important. For example, you may wish for your mentor to read through an abstract or manuscript, or you'd like to do a dry run of your PowerPoint presentation so you can get feedback. Send an agenda and materials to the mentor in advance (we recommend at least a week in advance, but this is something you should discuss with your mentor!), so that they can start thinking about things. Agendas will also help keep you on track. For example, if a mentor is particularly chatty or easily distracted, listing how much time during the

meeting you'd like to spend on each topic in the agenda helps redirect attention to tasks and avoids the discussion going off on a tangent.

3. **Bring your ideas:** You need to meet your mentor at the 50-yard line. Show what you have done, which ideas you considered, and share where you are stuck. Remind them where you left off and what you would like to do next. Your mentor wants to hear how you would approach a situation or challenge and, equally important, that you already started thinking. Instead of turning to your mentor as a blank canvas relying on them for every idea, write down one or two possible solutions and strategies, and ask your mentor to weigh in. Follow up with statements like these: "What am I missing or overlooking?" "What do you suggest I should do?" or "Given this, which way would you like me to proceed?" This not only shows your mentor that you took the initiative but also gives them an opportunity to help you fine-tune your approach. This small act has enormous potential as it helps you grow and refine your approach based on advice from your mentor.

4. **Keep your mentor informed:** When there is good news (a paper got accepted, you've been invited to present at a conference, etc.), you should see this as a team win and share it with your team! But especially when there is bad news (a grant was not discussed at study section, or someone has spotted a problem with your paper, resulting in a letter to the editor), you must be the first to share this with your mentor. Your mentor must know they can trust you, and you must show them that this is the case. Remember, they will find out anyway—better that it comes from you.

Make Meetings Efficient

If it's your first time meeting with your new mentor, you might be a bit nervous. That's to be expected as you want to make a good impression. Having discussion points is incredibly helpful and will guide the meeting. Don't overthink it or make it more complicated than it needs to be. Consider including the following topics during your meeting so that you can maximize productivity and efficiency and provide a fertile learning ground for both of you:

1. **Progress toward your goals:** Start by sharing updates since your last meeting, or if it's your first meeting, clearly outline your goals and proposed timelines to ensure agreement and alignment.

2. **Evaluating new opportunities:** Discuss any new projects you are contemplating and whether they align with your priorities. Be prepared to list the pros and cons for each.

3. **Overcoming roadblocks:** Provide a status update on any manuscripts or ongoing work, and highlight specific challenges where you need guidance. For example, you may be stuck with an analysis or struggling with a focus for the discussion section. These are items where having specifics to share with your mentor ahead of time can be very useful.

4. **Using your mentorship team:** Your primary mentor can help advise on how best to tap into your additional team members. Ask them how you should prepare for your team meetings—what makes the most sense and how best to use the team's time and the expertise of the group.

5. **Professional correspondence:** Review relevant correspondence with journal editors, grant program officers, or key stakeholders. Your mentor should know all that is happening with these individuals (they often know who they are on their own terms and can help you socialize your own relationship).

6. **Current projects and challenges:** Summarize what you're working on right now and any challenges you are facing. Be sure you receive actionable next steps.

7. **Networking opportunities:** Going to a meeting? Ask your mentor whom you should connect with and if they can introduce you to relevant contacts. Don't have a meeting or national conference on the radar? Ask them to define which conferences or events you should attend.

8. **Skill development:** Discuss areas where you want or need to grow and ask for recommendations on training, courses, webinars, or books. This is especially important if you are working on your career development grant or thinking about a new direction.

9. **Mentor's perspective:** Ask your mentor for feedback on how things are going, both in your work and in your mentoring relationship. Consider asking them, for example, if they recommend adjustments to the meeting schedule, agenda items, or frequency/type of communication.

Box 7.1 presents a sample email a mentor might appreciate before a meeting.

By following these meeting guidelines, you will find that lengthy conversations outside of the scheduled meeting are rarely necessary. You will also find yourself growing closer to your mentor and becoming more attuned to how best to optimize your time, effort, and focus. But, even with the best planning, time-sensitive issues sometimes arise that may require advice or approval from your mentor in order to move forward. When this occurs, be sure you have discussed the ideal method for getting in touch with your mentor (this is why hammering out these details in advance is helpful). Perhaps there is a key word in the subject line, or they prefer a text as a "heads up" to the longer

---

Box 7.1 Sample Email for Upcoming Mentoring Meeting

Subject: Agenda for Our Upcoming Mentoring Meeting

Dear [Mentor's Name],

Looking forward to our meeting on [Date]. Here's a brief agenda to keep us on track:

1. **Progress update:** Updates on my manuscript revisions for *JAMA* and the R01 grant submission.

2. **New opportunities:** Considering joining a multi-institutional research study on AI in diagnostics—thoughts?

3. **Challenges:** Struggling with IRB approval delays and balancing clinic time with research. Advice?

4. **Networking:** Would love an introduction to Dr. [Name] at [Institution] for collaboration on surgical outcomes research.

5. **Skill development:** Looking for leadership training opportunities in academic medicine. Any recommendations?

6. **Your feedback:** Any suggestions on improving my approach to career growth and time management?

Let me know if there's anything else you'd like to add. See you soon!

Best,
[Your Name]

---

email. Or they may just want you to call them. Either way, have a plan for when you need them on short notice and ensure you know what qualifies for such a call.

Most people are drowning in emails, and you certainly don't want a time-sensitive email to get lost. So be strategic in your communication. Be crystal clear in the subject line if this is urgent (and use that word sparingly). If you've ever seen the letters "TLDR," it stands for "too long, didn't read," and then offers a succinct summary. Start with that, in bold, followed by two to three brief sentences offering essential background. Then bold or highlight your question or action you need your mentor to take. The ideal questions are framed so they can be answered as quick "yes/no/let's discuss" options, which allows you to get what you need to move forward. Others use the BLUF approach: "bottom-line up-front." The point is the same: The first sentence or two should have the meat of the issue or question.

The BLUF for how we recommend communicating via email with your mentor is: A well-structured message makes it easier and faster for your mentor to respond, enabling them to answer easily and promptly from a mobile device.

Summary

Too often, the emphasis for quality mentorship is placed on the mentor, while the role of the mentee is overlooked. But the responsibility of the mentee is paramount. Like mentorship, menteeship is a practice that is honed over time. Highly effective mentees accelerate their careers by carefully selecting the right mentor and respectfully leveraging their mentor's expertise. Mentees must be ready, engaged, and proactive to benefit from their mentor's guidance.

Valuing your mentor's time, considering how and when communication occurs, preparing for meetings, and becoming highly organized are just a few key skills you will benefit from learning during your time being mentored. Acquiring these skills will help you achieve your goals and also make you a highly sought-after mentor in the future.

Take-Home Points

- As a mentee, you are responsible for driving the mentoring relationship forward. Make efficient use of the mentor's valuable time by preparing for meetings, providing an agenda, and communicating efficiently.
- Demonstrate your commitment and initiative by coming to meetings with specific challenges, having already invested effort into problem solving on your own, before seeking your mentor's instruction.
- Avoid overwhelming your mentor with disorganized thoughts, personal issues, or lengthy or excessive emails. When communicating outside of meeting times, use email in a way that allows mentors to provide "yes/no" answers to quickly reply.

8

Nine Things Standout Mentees Do

In healthcare, mentorship isn't just about learning the ropes or mastering the countless facts you've memorized and actualized over years of study. It's also about accelerating your growth, refining your skills, and making a lasting impact. As a mentee, you bring your own goals, work ethic, and personality to the table. Fortunately, you don't have to fundamentally change who you are to make the most of the experience. But not all mentees are created equal. There are certain qualities that set standout mentees apart, and knowing these qualities and adopting them will help you stand out. The best mentees don't just sit back and absorb; they engage, ask thoughtful questions, and take the initiative. For them, being mentored is not a passive task. It's one in which they are active participants. Whether you're a medical student shadowing a surgeon, a physician or nurse stepping into leadership, or a researcher developing specific knowledge and deep expertise in your area, the right approach can make the difference between success and failure.

Knowing What You Need

You need to have some clarity on what you need, where your strengths lie, and what areas you need to improve upon. Do you need help with skill development, career transitions, or leadership growth? Honesty begins with you, and the more vulnerable you are with yourself, the more you will know what to ask for. What are your professional goals? What is your mission? What do you want to be known for? What impact do you want to have on your field of study? And don't just think of impact in immediate terms—rather, start to think about your legacy. (It's never too early to start thinking about this.) With these ideas in mind, build a conversation with your mentor. Show your mentor that you're

DOI: 10.1201/9781003611233-10

invested in this mentoring relationship by crafting a written plan of your short- and long-term goals. Put both realistic and stretch goals on your list. And outline where you have strengths and where you need to grow.

Send the plan to your mentor in advance of your first meeting. While this might seem daunting, it serves multiple purposes. First, it helps you determine whether a shared vision of success exists. (Ideally, you should *both* be excited about *your* goals.) Second, it helps your mentor appropriately guide (and sponsor) you in a way that aligns with your goals. And third, it helps clarify roles and expectations for each of you. The upfront work can spare you disagreement (or worse, disappointment) later.

To ultimately prepare your current or potential mentor for this initial meeting, send (ideally several days before) a copy of your curriculum vitae (CV) and a one-page synopsis of your goals and aspirations. Be sure to also include a few sentences about your personal interests as the best conversations start with an alignment over a common thread. Are you a black belt in karate, can you code in different computer languages, play an instrument, or climb mountains? Or have you traveled the world, are you a first-generation immigrant or otherwise the product of a unique background? These are all good conversation starters that can help connect you to your mentor as a person. This background also helps when you meet with your mentor, as the conversation can quickly move to their thoughts about your future rather than pleasantries or time spent getting to know you. Your background, interests, and the way they're packaged all offer your mentor the opportunity to be more thoughtful if they want to take you on as a mentee. Even if they don't end up being your mentor, you will likely get helpful and thoughtful feedback since they will have mulled it over before meeting you. See Table 8.1 for a mentorship roadmap template, which can be used to clarify your mentorship goals and areas for growth.

Before Your First Meeting

From the very first meeting, you want to show your mentor that you are worth the investment of their time. After all, your success is their success . . . and they're looking for as close to a sure bet as they can get. To increase your chances of success, consider the following steps:

- **Do your homework:** Research your mentor's background, expertise, hobbies outside of work, and recent work. A little Googling goes a long way. Find out about prior mentees, and try to meet with them to learn

TABLE 8.1 Mentorship Roadmap Template

Section	Your Response	Examples
Short-Term Goals (6–12 months)		• Clinical research project • Training to improve bedside manner • Improve rounding efficiency
Long-Term Goals (3–5 years)		• Obtain a cardiology fellowship • Establish a mentorship program • Secure a new position
Preferred Mentorship Style		• Get big ideas from books and articles • Have discussions on book/article topics • Explore challenging ideas together
Key Skills to Develop		• Master a laparoscopic procedure • Develop healthcare leadership skills • Learn to use Stata®
Current Work and Challenges		• Work-life balance • Limited networking in specialty • Defining path for career opportunities
Preferred Type of Feedback		• Detailed case-based feedback • Real-time performance reviews • Written preferred over verbal
Measuring Ongoing Progress		• Give 1 presentation this academic year • Submit 2+ manuscripts to journals • Review 1–2 manuscripts (if invited)

more about their experiences. The more you know, the more productive your conversations will be.

- **Send materials in advance:** As discussed earlier (Chapter 7), sending your CV, goals, agenda, and other relevant material in advance gives the mentor time to mull over how they can best support you.

- **Prepare your introduction:** Yes, you already sent your material in advance, but a brief elevator pitch of who you are, your interests, and why you specifically sought them out as your mentor is ideal.

Structuring Your Meetings

As discussed in Chapter 7, it is helpful to send your mentor, in advance, an agenda, or list of topics to discuss in the meeting. In our experience, it is best to focus on no more than two to four key topics for the discussion. If you have a 30-minute meeting, give each topic 10 minutes. If you have 40 minutes and two topics, give them 20 each. Budget your time wisely to set up the meeting for success. It helps keep it on track and focused. Similarly, you may find it helpful to use a personal tracking sheet that you update after each meeting. See Table 8.2 for a template. We provide this as an example and leave it to the individual mentee to determine whether it is useful. Track each mentoring meeting using a table as in this example.

TABLE 8.2 Sample Mentorship Meeting Tracking Sheet

Topic	✓	Key Points Discussed	Next Steps	Due By
Review recent patient case studies and discuss diagnostic decision making	☐			
Strategies for balancing clinical responsibilities with research	☐			
Networking strategies for career advancement in healthcare	☐			
Implementation of a new workflow for patient consultations	☐			
Draft of research manuscript for submission	☐			
Time management between clinical and academic duties	☐			
Develop a plan for presenting research at a medical conference	☐			
Create teaching scripts for learners	☐			
Prepare and present a Grand Rounds lecture	☐			
Compose an interview guide for hiring a project manager, research associate, or statistician	☐			
Read a book on how to have difficult conversations with direct reports	☐			
Learn how to review financial reports to track revenue and expenses (e.g., clinical)	☐			
Ensure adequate time for family and self-care	☐			

Key Takeaways

Navigating Mentorship across Career Phases

It is often said, "What got you here, won't get you there."[1] It's also true that *who* got you here may not get you there. As your career evolves, so do your mentoring needs. If you spoke to your PhD mentor daily or weekly as you were progressing with your research, your needs when you are a postdoc or junior faculty member will be quite different, so you will need different people for guidance. If you are becoming a chief or chair, you don't need the same type of mentoring you did as a junior faculty member. It's not rude to approach different mentors throughout your career; it's the right thing to do. Ideally, you've thought about this and have a mentorship team that is scaled for this growth. After all, mentorship is not a life sentence.

Early Career (Students, Trainees, Residents, and Fellows)

At this stage of your career, you are building your foundation and your skills and starting to define your network. Take every opportunity you can to learn and be around those who want to teach you. Your primary goal here is to develop a solid foundation of knowledge and clinical and research know-how. As you see patients in the clinic or on the wards, scrub into surgeries, or deliver babies, this is when you learn the importance of teamwork in healthcare. This is no time to be shy about asking questions or diving deep. No one expects you to know everything (or much), so ask away. This is also the time to develop your EQ (emotional quotient) and interpersonal skills[2,3] (what used to be known as soft skills). Learn how to communicate skillfully, relate to others effectively, and develop a reputation as being curious, reliable, and a team player. You typically only have one chance to make a strong first impression[4] as a clinician, researcher, administrator, or healthcare leader; this is the time to lay that strong foundation for your future.

Mid-Career (Attendings, Practicing Professionals, and Early Leadership Roles)

In medical, nursing, and other healthcare professional schools, leadership development is usually not part of the formal curriculum. There is a lot of learning by observing and learning by doing[5-7] that occur in leadership development in healthcare. But the truth is that you are leading most of the time—leading your patients through their healthcare journeys, your medical team when you are on service, and yourself through the trials and tribulations of academia. If you want to stand out, ask your mentor to recommend leadership development courses, seminars, and programs you should attend. Or better yet, find open/free ones on your campus or those of others (virtual options work just fine), and make the time to attend.

Develop Your Second Lane

You will always be known for your clinical, educational, or research strengths, but as a leader, you need a second lane. Something that you are passionate about and willing to take a stand on, and eventually be known for. Some examples include successful insurance/payer negotiations, grant writing, patient safety, burnout/well-being, financial savvy, communication skills, humanism in healthcare, procedural coaching, and how the three authors of this book found each other: mentoring. This will help you develop your niche area beyond your clinical or research expertise. There will always be someone more knowledgeable on your clinical or research topic, but you are often the expert in the room on the topic of your second lane. Combined with your clinical, educational, or research background, this second lane often opens new doors for you.

At this point in your career, finding a sponsor is essential. You need to find people who can tell you what doors (opportunities) exist, open the doors for you, and mentor you so that you can succeed as you walk through those doors. Finding a sponsor need not be hard. Your mentor or mentorship team can help introduce you to those who are higher up in the organizational chart (either at your organization or a different one) who can advocate on your behalf. Remember, it's better to make a friend before you need one! Knowing someone before you ask them to sponsor you can easily make them more willing to say yes.

Late Career (Senior Leaders and Developing Your Legacy)

As you advance in your career, you will be known for many things. But you will be remembered for those you mentored, sponsored, or coached. The more senior you become, the more you will be asked to mentor others. Think about how you can support and develop the next generation of healthcare providers and how you can develop the time, energy, and space for this activity. Is it time to pivot from one-to-one mentoring to a group model so that you can scale your efforts? Or are you better as a sponsor than a mentor, given your many commitments? Certainly, this has changed for Vineet, who is now the chair of a large department and doesn't have as much time for one-to-one mentoring. However, group sessions and serving as a sponsor are much easier to achieve.

Realize that it's lonely at the top. If you become a division chief, chair, or dean, you are often shielded from the raw truth, given your position and influence. Your previous group of confidantes now report to you, and there are implications to what they say and how they say it. The dynamics have fundamentally changed. That's why even those at the top of the field need mentors[8] to bounce ideas off of, coaches to help them manage through various challenges, and others to tell the unvarnished truth.

Dr. J. Randall Curtis, a palliative care leader who died of amyotrophic lateral sclerosis in February 2023, and someone whom Sanjay had the privilege of learning from, once said:

> Before my diagnosis, I used to think of my legacy as the papers I had published and the impact that my research has had on the field of medicine. Since my diagnosis, my thinking has changed. I now see my legacy as the people I have mentored and helped mentor and the people that they have mentored. This vision of legacy gives me much more joy and happiness than my old vision of legacy.[9]

Even at the top, it's the meaningful connections with mentors and mentees that continue to matter.

Am I an Effective Mentee?

Being an effective mentee requires work beyond just showing up for meetings. As we discussed in Chapter 7, it is the mentee's responsibility to drive the meetings, select the topics to be discussed, pinpoint where they need help, and follow up and share with the mentor what was tried, what wasn't, and why.[10] These types of activities as a mentee shows you are an active, not passive participant in this mentoring relationship. After all, if you are not invested, why should your mentor be?

Show, don't tell. If you want your mentor to see you are innovative, hardworking, and dependable, prove it; don't say it. Growth mindset, where you are open to feedback and see it as an opportunity for enhancement, not critique, is pivotal.[11] Remember, feedback is a gift. It's much easier for your mentor to say, "This looks good," than to provide detailed edits to a work product. Tracked changes and extensive rewrites or comments can be intimidating and make you feel defeated, but they are a sign of a mentor who cares. Here are some things to keep in mind as you pave your way to success.

Keep Your Mentor in the Loop

A mentor can't help you if you're not being forthcoming with your efforts and what you're attempting to achieve. Smoke and mirrors, vague or broad descriptions of your activities and endeavors will frustrate your mentor. Remember, your mentor likely knows many people. The last thing you want is for them to hear about your involvement in something or a negative outcome from someone else—especially if it distracts from your responsibilities or differs from what they expected you to be working on. Whenever you are taking on new tasks or those that are tangential to your stated goals, we highly recommend checking with your mentor. Keep them in the loop.

Be Open about Obstacles

Challenges and mistakes are part of the process, and your mentor is well aware of this. Remember, they too were once a mentee, and they too made mistakes. However, your mentor is not a mind reader. If you don't discuss your worries or errors with them, you're losing a prime opportunity to learn problem-solving, management, or coping skills.

Sometimes, we can't see the forest from the trees. Every problem seems insurmountable. Even in these situations, your mentor can help you climb out. They are more familiar with this terrain than you are. Get comfortable bringing up issues large and small. Questions or comments ranging from "I'm completely overwhelmed" to "I've been accused of plagiarism or scientific misconduct" should all be discussed with your mentor. They have the benefit of perspective. Remember, it is rare that a seasoned mentor will be caught off guard by something you tell them.

Listen More Than You Talk

You have two ears and one mouth—use them at that ratio. You are meeting with the mentor so that you can learn and grow. That's hard to do if you are monopolizing the conversation and not giving yourself space to learn. Evaluate your "TLR," or talking-to-listening ratio. The goal? Ensure it's less than 1. When you are not listening, you are not learning.[12] Practice the art of not interrupting. Having an agenda certainly helps accomplish this goal. Consciously pay attention to when you are inclined to interrupt and force yourself to pause until your mentor has concluded speaking.

Be Professional

While one would hope this is obvious, it bears repeating. The mentoring relationship is no place for drama, complaining, or gossiping. While emotions indicate passion and enthusiasm, everything has limits, and you don't want to create patterns. Frequent emotional outbursts can rapidly tarnish your reputation. And remember, the purpose of your meeting with your mentor is to grow your abilities, not to be defensive. Of course, you should ask questions and understand the rationale for recommendations or feedback. But avoid the knee-jerk response to rationalize or disagree with the guidance you are getting. Listen to what is being said with care and intent. It's for your own good.

Finish What You Start

Be the person people can depend on. No matter how minor, when you say you'll do something, do it. Having things fall through the cracks is infuriating to everyone who was counting on you. Develop a process for tracking all your tasks and promised to-do's, and check regularly to be sure you're not letting anything slip. (See Chapter 7 for a tracking sheet example.) If you know you are going to be late on something, let your mentor know that will be the case and let them know why. There are often good reasons—and your mentor will understand. But only if you let them know and don't make a habit of not following through. The bottom line: Develop a reputation as a closer.

It's Not All about You

Healthcare and science is a team sport. Learn to generously and graciously give others credit where and when it is due. Developing a reputation as a team player will enhance your chances of being included in future group opportunities that contribute to your professional growth. Lose the "me" mentality; it pays dividends in the long run. Helping out—even a little bit—goes a long way. Remember, your mentor gets paid exactly $0 to help you. If they can do it for you, so can you for someone else.

Under-Promise and Over-Deliver

Your action (and inaction) reflect on you and your abilities. Always put forth your best work and give yourself ample time to do it so you don't miss deadlines. However long you think it will take you to finish a job,

Instructions: Score yourself from 1 (never) to 5 (always) on each question.

TABLE 8.3 Periodic Self-Assessment

Evaluation Question	1	2	3	4	5
Do I clearly communicate my goals to my mentor?					
Do I take the initiative in setting up meetings and following up?					
Am I receptive to constructive feedback?					
Do I keep my mentor updated on my progress and challenges?					
Am I actively applying my mentor's advice?					
Do I express gratitude and respect for my mentor's time?					

triple the time estimate. Best to ask for more than the time you think you need to do a job well and try to finish ahead of schedule. Strive to be the mentee who under-promises and over-delivers—the one who sets realistic expectations and consistently exceeds them. Building this reputation will benefit you in the long run. The opposite—over-promising while under-delivering, making grandiose promises but failing to follow through—can derail careers. We all remember the mentees who were good at this!

Periodically self-assess to gauge where you stand and identify areas for improvement. Consider the self-assessment in Table 8.3 to get you started, see where you excel, and accept where you can use improvement.

Summary of Nine Things Standout Mentees Do

The best mentees don't just absorb knowledge—they engage, take initiative, and drive the relationship forward. Here's what sets standout mentees apart:

1. **Take ownership of your mentoring experience:** You are responsible for calling and driving meetings, setting topics, and following up. If you're not invested, why should your mentor be?
2. **Show, don't tell:** Demonstrate your dedication through action. A growth mindset helps you turn feedback into progress.
3. **Keep your mentor in the loop:** Be transparent about your efforts and challenges. Vague or broad updates frustrate mentors.
4. **Be open about obstacles:** Mistakes and struggles are learning opportunities. The more honest you are, the more your mentor can help.
5. **Listen more than you talk:** You have two ears and one mouth—use them accordingly. Avoid monopolizing the conversation.

6. **Be professional:** No drama, gossip, or complaining. Approach mentorship with positivity and a solutions-oriented mindset.

7. **Finish what you start:** Do what you say you will. Being reliable strengthens trust and respect in the mentorship.

8. **It's not all about you:** A mentorship thrives on reciprocity. Give credit where it's due, and support those around you.

9. **Under-promise and over-deliver:** Set realistic expectations, meet deadlines, and aim to exceed expectations whenever possible.

Summary

Being a great mentee does not mean you have to change who you are or fit yourself into a cookie cutter mold. People of all different personalities, work styles, and convictions achieve their goals while keeping their personal values at the center—they often become outstanding mentors later in their career as well.

But you can always adopt good habits to better promote your growth. Mentees should remain authentic, embracing their individuality while adding those qualities that distinguish standout mentees—such as actively engaging, listening more than talking, asking insightful questions, and taking initiative. Establishing these solid practices for productivity early in your career will help you ensure you're always putting your best self forward. Learn from those around you who have mentored for years. There is a reason they've gotten to where they are.

Take-Home Points

- Rather than changing who you are, leverage your unique strengths and individuality while adopting effective habits from mentors.
- Be a person of your word. Whether a small task or a major one, do what you say you will do, and do it well. Under-promise and over-deliver, show your dedication through action, and communicate when you face obstacles.
- Your mentoring needs will change through different stages in your career. Seek diverse mentors on your team who can provide relevant guidance and opportunities as your professional journey progresses.

9

Beware of the Mentee Landmines

Ruth was asked to mentor a medical student. She had a specific project the student could work on that would have resulted in a first-authored, peer-reviewed publication in a biomedical journal. This was ideal work for a student who was trying to enhance their curriculum vitae (CV) before applying for residency. The problems surfaced on day one.

The student never showed up on the first day, citing that his calendar didn't sync. The red flags continued as Ruth noticed that every draft and outline he submitted to her was written—not simply enhanced—by artificial intelligence (AI). When she told him he needs to read articles, not just have AI summarize them, he asked if there was any other faster way. Finally, one day in the early afternoon, he told her that he was leaving midday because he was tired and going home to take a nap. Ruth was frustrated at the lack of initiative, repetitive and often unethical shortcuts, and lack of professionalism. Ruth realized she could not help someone succeed until they were ready to do the work.

In her book, *Right Kind of Wrong*, Harvard Business School professor Dr. Amy Edmondson emphasizes that not all failures are created equal.[1] She refers to two types of failures: The bad kind, which are preventable, and the good kind, which you can learn from and may lead to important discoveries. The intelligent failures, those that are a result of exploring a new territory, are good. The basic failures, those that are preventable and due to inattention, neglect, or overconfidence, are bad.

Despite the best of intentions, there are always times when a mentee makes mistakes.[2] If they are intelligent failures, that's okay, as those can be

 DOI: 10.1201/9781003611233-11

learning opportunities. (In fact, many scientific discoveries have resulted from such failures.) It's when preventable mistakes are made, or worse yet, a pattern of such egregious errors emerges—such as those by Ruth's medical student—that problems start to percolate.

Satya Nadella, the CEO of Microsoft, said it best when he encouraged his employees to be a "learn it all," not a "know it all." A sensible mentee is always aiming to be mature, responsible, and ambitious. They are always looking to learn new things, try new collaborations, or follow a new path as guided by their mentor or mentorship team. Unfortunately, some otherwise good mentees become overly absorbed in appearances, desiring to look like experts from the start of their journey—before they actually know anything. Obsessing over your purported image isn't just pointless; it can set you up for some serious missteps. We call these preventable errors "mentee landmines"—and offer a path along this treacherous road.

The Most Common Mentee Landmines and How to Avoid Them

Successfully navigating mentoring relationships (and fulfilling your career potential) require more than just ambition—they demand strategic decision making and self-awareness. Too many mentees, eager to prove themselves, make critical errors and fall into patterns that can derail their growth, and/ or strain their relationships with their mentors. After all, a mentor can clean up your mess only so many times. Here are some of the most common missteps mentees make and some practical strategies to avoid them.

Saying "Yes" to Everything: The Overcommitted Mentee

Often the reward for good work is, well, more work. That's fine as you want to be a team player. But be careful not to become the mentee who says yes to every collaborative project, paper, or presentation. You will quickly end up overcommitted. First and foremost, learn to say "no" politely. Being a "yes person" early in your career is important, but you must be strategic about what you will versus will not do. Saying yes to everything or everyone will not do anyone, including yourself, any favors. Always discuss opportunities with your mentor and your mentorship team to ensure you don't commit to projects that aren't aligned with your goals or career. Overextending yourself will ultimately result in lower-quality work product and a tarnished reputation. Once your reputation is damaged, it's hard to bounce back.

There is an art to saying "no" to things that may not be value-adding for you. We often use the framework from William Ury's book, *The Power of a Positive No.*[3] First, consider if "no" is an option; depending on your organization and your boss, it may not be. If your boss is the editor-in-chief of a major journal, and he asks you to review a manuscript, no matter how busy you are, it's probably in your best interest to do it. However, if you have autonomy to choose, be more discerning. If you are asked to do something that appears to be a major time sink, ask yourself whether the assignment aligns with your immediate and long-term goals. And bring this to your mentor for a discussion to make sure you're reading the situation and opportunity correctly. By saying "no" to one thing, you are saying "yes" to something else—usually yourself.

Second, be sincere yet straightforward when turning down the extra work: "Thank you for the offer, but at this critical stage in my career I will need to focus on X" (your goals and priorities, such as writing a career development grant or a peer-reviewed paper) ". . . and this project will distract me from that goal." If you have discussed this with your mentor (which we hope you have), another effective way to politely bow out could be, "I would love to be able to do this, but I don't have much time now, and my mentor would like me to focus on my primary projects."

The final point is saying "yes" to the relationship. You don't want to create enemies or leave people with a sour taste in their mouth. So it is important to end the conversation with a pleasant and cooperative tone. One way to do this is to recommend someone else for the opportunity, especially if you know they may be interested. For example: "Even though I can't assist you now given my looming grant deadline (or insert other priorities here), please let me know if I can suggest someone else for this project who is equally capable (or give them the name of a person who you think will be great). Or another way is to propose that you could reconsider when/ if your load becomes a little easier to manage. For example: "When I do come up for air in six months, I'd love to reconnect and think about how to work together on this or related projects."

The Confidence Trap: Balancing Self-Reliance with Asking for Help

Nobody wants to be micromanaged, and busy mentors really don't have the time or interest to approve or sign off on everything that you do. They want you to learn to be independent and are preparing you for that stage of your career. You should certainly keep your mentor in the loop, but when the mentoring relationship is grounded in trust, you can and should be able to proceed with various projects without your mentor's explicit blessing.

You are still learning, so you won't have all the answers. In fact, you don't know what you don't know. Giving incorrect and poorly thought-out answers or making impulsive decisions is not likely to serve you (or your mentor) well. Ideally, you and your mentor have discussed how much latitude you may have in various areas. In healthcare, knowing when to seek guidance from your mentor can be the difference between a well-informed decision and a costly mistake. While independence is the goal, no one gets behind the wheel of a car without practice. Recognize that there are key moments when asking for guidance is not only beneficial but essential. And while there may be standard protocols for many things, sometimes there are no clear answers. This is no different in clinical care—for example, when a critically ill patient is not responding to vasopressors, and several differential diagnoses are possible. Any attending physician will appreciate that discussion, and, yes, so will you because you will learn and grow. A mentee should thus know when they are out of their depth and when to ask for backup.

Poor Communication: The Silent Career Killer

If you don't know, ask for help. That's a sound rule to go by. Don't hesitate to ask for your mentor's perspective or assistance when you think it would be helpful. After all, that's part of what a good mentor (and mentee) should do. If it's a simple question where you are just looking for reassurance, a quick two- to three-sentence email with background and a "yes/no" reply is often all you need (as discussed in Chapter 7). Noting on the top of the email in bold that you only need a yes/no response or if the email is just a FYI and no action is needed is also helpful. If the issue is more complex, save it for a face-to-face meeting. These meetings provide the ideal opportunity to address your questions and nuanced issues in greater depth. And by now, you've learned how to plan for these by sending an agenda and background information ahead of time and ensuring that there will be sufficient time for the discussion.

Good mentoring requires good communication. No mentoring relationship can thrive—or even survive—without open, honest dialogue. Learn to communicate clearly and efficiently so that there are no lingering questions about what is happening, what the next step is, and where you are heading. If you aren't clear on what is being recommended or what the next action steps are, pause the conversation and ask for clarification *before* committing to anything. Another important action is to summarize what was discussed to ensure you understood correctly. Maintaining this type of clear and open communication helps ensure that both you and your mentor are on the same wavelength.

"Ghosting" your mentor—disappearing without communication—never ends well. It sets off red flags and flares. After a momentary panic for your well-being, it quickly erodes trust, and damages your reputation (especially if you've been busy doing things they don't know about). Mentors invest their time and effort into guiding you. When you go silent, it signals a lack of respect. Consistent communication, even if it is just to provide a brief update or acknowledge a delay, helps maintain trust and keeps the mentoring relationship healthy and strong.

Lack of Honesty and Accountability

As previously mentioned, intelligent mistakes are a natural part of mentee-ship. They are a golden opportunity to reflect and grow. These types of errors are expected. When this happens (and it will), be truthful and honest. If after every mistake you blame others, resent constructive criticism, or make excuses for half-baked or tardy work, it is time to look in the mirror. After all, it can't always be everyone else's fault.

Research has shown that when a workplace is psychologically safe, and people don't feel there would be retaliation for making errors, they are more likely to report them and learn from the experience.[4] When you make a mistake, admit it, and develop strategies to avoid similar errors in the future. Once is excusable; twice (or more often) is a pattern. Your honesty and willingness to admit fault will be welcomed. Hoping it won't get noticed or avoiding your mentor (ghosting), will not help you or the situation. It will only make it worse. Ultimately, your mentor will discover what you've been (or haven't been) doing, and both your relationship and your career may suffer.

We can't reiterate this enough: If there are obstacles to moving your work forward, talk to your mentor sooner rather than later. A good mentor will never fault you for not making progress if they are made aware of what the legitimate barriers are. But you will be to blame if you don't keep them informed.

Mistakes are inevitable, but how you handle them can define your professional trajectory. Owning your mistakes with honesty, accountability, and a growth mindset serves to preserve your credibility and strengthen your mentor's trust in you. Box 9.1 outlines how to turn setbacks into opportunities for growth.

Box 9.1 Strategies for Owning Mistakes and Turning Them into Career Growth Moments

1. **Acknowledge the Mistake Quickly and Transparently**

   - Avoid making excuses or placing blame on others. Instead, take responsibility as soon as you recognize the error by acknowledging what you could have done differently.

   - Example: If you misinterpret research data and present incorrect findings, acknowledge the mistake immediately rather than waiting for someone else to point it out. It doesn't matter if the analyst you worked with did it wrong, or there was an error in the code: You own the work; the buck stops with you. The best thing to do when you get something wrong is to get it right and be transparent and prompt about it.

2. **Analyze What Went Wrong**

   - Reflect on the root cause of the mistake and discuss it with your mentor. Was it a lack of knowledge, miscommunication, or rushing through a task?

   - In the previous example, perhaps you're not spending enough time with your analyst or looking at the actual statistical code to understand what is being done.

3. **Develop a Corrective Plan**

   - Show initiative by outlining a plan to fix the mistake and prevent it from happening again. Keeping with our example, resolve to spend time looking at the raw output or working hand in hand with your statistician going forward.

4. **Seek Constructive Feedback**

   - Use the mistake as a learning opportunity by asking your mentor for advice on improving your approach. For example, how may you tell your analyst that what they did was incorrect? How can you work better with them going forward? What are some warning signs you should be looking for when examining the regression outputs?

5. **Demonstrate Growth over Time**

   - Implement the lessons learned, and show your mentor that you've applied their guidance in future work. Bring the raw code and output with you the next time or ensure you double-/triple-check the tables against the regression output to verify accuracy. Set up a process going forward so this doesn't happen again.

By being professional and transparent when handling mistakes, and having a solutions-focused attitude, mentees can turn challenges into pivotal learning experiences that propel their careers forward.

The Exploitive Mentor: Recognizing and Handling Mentorship Malpractice

As discussed in Chapter 4, while rare, some mentors assign mentees busy-work or give them projects unrelated to their interests or goals. We call these mentors "exploiters"—they torpedo their mentees and see them as task-doers rather than future leaders. They are prioritizing efficiency over development. Exploiters value managers, not scientists or creative thinkers. Then there are the "hijackers"—mentors who take credit for a mentee's idea, sometimes going as far as claiming first- or senior-author spots on manuscripts without doing any of the heavy lifting. Worse, some may submit a mentee's ideas or preliminary data in grants without proper attribution. Unfortunately, these stories aren't rare in the scientific community, so make sure to recognize and address these behaviors early. (Chapter 10 discusses ways you can address these.) This is also why speaking to former mentees can be helpful!

Whether making an error or dealing with misappropriated contributions to work, difficult conversations with your mentor shouldn't be avoided. Your mentor is there to help you. If you keep things bottled up, it will only get you more upset and start to cloud your judgment. See Table 9.1 for some scripts we prepared to help you get started.

TABLE 9.1 Ten Common Healthcare Scenarios and Suggested Scripts for Navigating Difficult Conversations with Your Mentor

Scenario	Suggested Script
Receiving Excessive Administrative Tasks	"I appreciate the opportunities you've provided. I've noticed that a significant portion of my time is spent on administrative tasks, and that limits my ability to focus on my clinical and research development. Could we discuss how I can contribute in a way that aligns better with my training goals?"
Being Assigned Work outside of Specialty	"Thank you for trusting me with these responsibilities. I wanted to discuss some recent assignments that fall outside my area of focus. While I'm eager to learn, I'd love to explore how I can balance these with projects that align more closely with my interests. Would you be open to discussing this?"

(Continued)

TABLE 9.1 (Continued)

Scenario	Suggested Script
Needing More Hands-On Clinical Experience	"I truly appreciate all your mentorship. I've realized that while I'm gaining valuable theoretical knowledge, I would benefit from more hands-on clinical exposure. Would it be possible to get involved in more procedural cases or direct patient care under your supervision?"
Handling Ethical Concerns in Patient Care	"I recently encountered a situation that raised ethical concerns for me, and I'd really value your perspective. A patient's family requested to withhold a diagnosis, and I'm struggling with how to navigate the balance between patient autonomy and family wishes. How would you recommend handling this?"
Not Receiving Enough Feedback	"I really value your guidance and would love to improve my skills. I've noticed that I don't always receive feedback on my performance, though. Would you be open to providing structured feedback on a consistent basis so I can work on areas that need improvement?"
Balancing Research and Clinical Duties	"I'm committed to both my clinical responsibilities and my research, but I'm finding it challenging to manage both effectively. I'd love to hear any advice you have on prioritization and time management. Could we discuss strategies to ensure success in both areas?"
Mentor Taking Credit for Work	"I'm grateful for all the support and opportunities I've had. I wanted to bring up something sensitive—on a recent project, I noticed my contributions weren't fully acknowledged. I want to ensure we're aligned on proper credit for our work. Could we discuss how to handle this moving forward?"
Unclear Expectations for Career Progression	"I appreciate all the mentorship you've provided. I'm trying to get a clearer sense of the steps I should be taking for my career progression, and I'd love your insight into milestones I should be aiming for. Could we set up a time to discuss this?"
Struggling with Workload and Burnout	"I'm truly grateful for all the opportunities I've been given. That said, I've been feeling overwhelmed by my workload and worry that it might be affecting the quality of my work. Do you have any advice on how I can manage my responsibilities more effectively while maintaining a healthy balance?"
Handling a Conflict with a Colleague	"I've encountered a professional challenge that I could use some guidance on. I've been having difficulties collaborating with a colleague, and I want to make sure I handle it professionally. Have you dealt with similar situations, and how would you recommend approaching it?"

Summary

Mistakes will be made when mentees are early in their career (and they still happen later in your career too). However, a good number of mistakes are common and can be avoided. Implement strategies to avoid common pitfalls, like overcommitting, communicating poorly, or failing to take responsibility for your mistakes.

Honesty and accountability are essential for turning mistakes into learning opportunities. Openly acknowledge and analyze mistakes, demonstrating your willingness to grow. And when you feel you are struggling, talk to your mentor sooner rather than later. They are there to help you.

Take-Home Points

- Mistakes are inevitable, but you can avoid the most common ones. Embrace the mistakes you do make as learning opportunities, and use them to plan for improvement.
- Keep open lines of communication with your mentor, especially when facing issues. Alerting them about issues early on can prevent problems from escalating and will strengthen your relationship by demonstrating trust and transparency.
- Cultivate the right balance between confidence and humility by discerning when to ask for help. If you feel your mentor is exploiting you, address your concerns openly, and consider ending the mentorship if necessary.

10

Moving On from a Mentoring Relationship: Knowing When It's Time

If you've done things right, you will have absorbed much from your mentor and learned most of what they can give you. You've also had a mentoring team you have worked with and have realized the value of diverse views while benefiting from the skills uniquely distributed across people. As you grow, it is thus inevitable that your needs will change. And the skills you now need are different. In other words, what got you here may not get you to the next rung of the ladder.

A mentoring relationship can end when a mentee meets their goals, graduates, or goes in a new leadership or research direction. Think of medical/graduate students, residents, and fellows. Or of a faculty member who gets their first independent grant and wants to start their own program of inquiry. These are natural times when separating from a mentor makes sense.

On the other hand, it may be that you are not getting what you need from your mentorship team. Or worse, that your mentor is not supporting but rather hindering your progress. In these situations, it may be time to get other help or, in the most serious cases, walk away.

Both of these scenarios require ending relationships with your mentors and moving on to new ones. In Chapter 4 we introduce the concept of mentorship malpractice and the various phenotypes of active and passive mentorship malpractice. But in this chapter—since it is geared toward the mentee—we focus on arming the mentee to address the situation.

Problematic Mentor Behaviors

Sadly, mentorship can fail if the mentor creates problems. The worst is due to negligent behavior from a mentor, such as those discussed in Chapter 4. These types of egregious behaviors must be addressed immediately (see the scripts in Chapter 9). If you allow an unproductive or toxic mentorship to persist, you jeopardize your career.

As discussed in Chapter 4, there are red flag tormentor behaviors, which you need to be aware of:

- Taking credit for mentee's work;
- Being overly possessive of mentee's growth;
- Avoiding conflict or responsibility;
- Lack of availability;
- Exploiting mentee for personal gain.

These mentors, ranging from the hijacker to the exploiter, possessor, bottleneck, country clubber, and world traveler, will derail your growth and lead to plummeting self-confidence. Use the checklist found in Table 10.1 to identify potential mentorship malpractice and determine whether your mentor is derailing your career.

TABLE 10.1 Is Your Mentor Helping or Hindering Your Growth?

Tormentor	Consideration	Healthcare Example
The Hijacker *Takes credit for your work and diminishes your contributions.*	Does your mentor fail to acknowledge your contributions in research, projects, or publications? ☐ Yes ☐ No	Your mentor lists themselves as first author on a paper on which you did most of the work.
	Is proper credit excluded or forgotten when your mentor discusses your project with others? ☐ Yes ☐ No	Your mentor has another trainee present your case at a conference without mentioning your role in the work.
	Does your mentor overshadow your achievements rather than raise your visibility? ☐ Yes ☐ No	Your mentor takes credit for your ideas as their own during meetings with others.

(Continued)

TABLE 10.1 (Continued)

Tormentor	Consideration	Healthcare Example
The Exploiter *Assigns tasks that benefit them but do not help you grow.*	Are the projects assigned to you out of line with your career development trajectory? ☐ Yes ☐ No	Instead of clinical research opportunities, your mentor asks you to proofread their new book.
	Do you end up with menial tasks rather than learning opportunities? ☐ Yes ☐ No	You are asked to handle clerical work instead of engaging in meaningful projects.
	Does the work feel like it helps your mentor's career more than yours? ☐ Yes ☐ No	Your mentor assigns you to collect data for their study even though you need to do the same for your own project.
The Possessor *Isolates you from chances to collaborate with others.*	Does your mentor interfere with or prevent you from seeking advice from other mentors or professionals? ☐ Yes ☐ No	Your mentor discourages you from forming a mentorship team or working with other faculty.
	Are you discouraged from attending external conferences, workshops, or training? ☐ Yes ☐ No	Your mentor insists that all your work stays with their research group and refuses to let you present independently.
	Does your mentor limit rather than support your networking efforts? ☐ Yes ☐ No	Your mentor does not introduce you to key figures in the field, even when obvious opportunities arise.
The Bottleneck *Slows your progress with missed deadlines, no feedback, or delayed decision making.*	Do you receive feedback in a way that slows your progress? ☐ Yes ☐ No	Your mentor takes weeks to review your manuscript, delaying submission and reducing your productivity.
	Is it difficult to get a response from your mentor when you ask for help? ☐ Yes ☐ No	Your mentor submits your residency recommendation letter after the deadline, delaying your application processing.
	Does your mentor regularly miss project deadlines or fail to provide sufficient support? ☐ Yes ☐ No	You need IRB approval for your research study, but your mentor delays signing off on the protocol you want to submit.

(Continued)

TABLE 10.1 (Continued)

Tormentor	Consideration	Healthcare Example
The Country Clubber *Avoids difficult conversations and provides minimal guidance.*	Does your mentor provide flattery instead of constructive feedback to help you improve? ☐ Yes ☐ No	Your mentor only gives vague, positive comments like, "You're doing great!" without specific guidance on a given task.
	Do they avoid addressing challenges and conflicts rather than facing tough conversations? ☐ Yes ☐ No	You express concerns about a difficult team dynamic, but your mentor changes the subject whenever you do.
	Is your mentor disconnected from your professional development? ☐ Yes ☐ No	Your mentor uses meeting times to socialize with you, rather than providing support and advice on your career.
The World Traveler *Frequently unavailable and unresponsive.*	Is your mentor often unavailable when you need guidance? ☐ Yes ☐ No	Your mentor is always traveling for speaking engagements. You can only schedule occasional meetings with them.
	Does your mentor frequently cancel regular check-in meetings? ☐ Yes ☐ No	Inevitably as your one-on-one meetings approach, your mentor will cancel or reschedule.
	Is your mentor disengaged from your progress? ☐ Yes ☐ No	Your mentor has not bothered to check in on your research progress for months.

Next Steps

- If you answered "Yes" to multiple questions, your mentor may be hindering your growth. Reflect on whether this mentoring relationship is still serving your goals.
- Consider discussing your concerns with your mentor or with your entire mentorship team when you meet next.
- If the mentoring relationship is no longer beneficial, start considering new mentorship opportunities.
- For severe issues such as exploitation, credit theft, or ethical violations, seek guidance from trusted colleagues, institutional leadership, or human resources.
- Remember, mentorship should be a mutually beneficial relationship—if it is hindering your success, it may be time to transition professionally.

A word of caution to mentees: Nothing will improve if you let these behaviors fester. They will not disappear on their own, no matter how hard you wish for that to be the case. There is no easy way to say this. If a mentor is inattentive or spiteful with their power, you expose yourself to personal and professional downfall. What happens thereafter could adversely affect your career.

Strategies for Navigating a Troubled Mentorship

If you feel you are the victim of mentorship malpractice, start document-ing the interactions, save the emails, and engage your mentorship team about what you are observing or experiencing. The sooner you do this, the better. If it is early in the process, it may be salvageable. The longer you wait, the more toxic it becomes, and the harder it is to break the cycle. Communicating what you are experiencing is a must. Chapter 9 (Table 9.1) presents scripts for navigating difficult conversations with your mentor.

Be an Upstander, Not a Bystander

Every menial task given by the exploiter or missed first-authored paper sto-len by the hijacker must have limits and consequences, respectively. Sure, mentees need to be an active team member and pitch in, but they shouldn't only be doing menial roles. With the help of their mentorship team (which we will discuss), mentees must put their foot down and insist on a change. Deciding not to take action is a choice and is usually a mistake. Even if there is fear of retribution, the chances are you, the mentee, won't be worse off than you are now, and you will have taken back your power.

Speak Up for Yourself

Effective communication starts with clarity and is the thoroughfare for pre-venting mentorship malpractice. This is especially necessary and important when dealing with passive mentorship malpractice. With the more active ones, the mentee, with guidance from their mentoring team (or a coach or another more senior individual), must commit and communicate clear bound-aries (e.g., I can't stay at work after 6 PM, I am not able to babysit your children, I really am not comfortable submitting that human subjects application for you as I am not part of that project) and speak up when a violation occurs. Mistakes happen, but if they become a pattern, the cycle should be broken.

Establish a Mentoring Team

A mentoring team can offer new perspectives, expand your network, and help you deal with toxic mentors. Having a team where you can surface issues can help deal with the problematic behavior and implement remedies. If these are not helpful, the team can help you gracefully exit a bad mentoring relationship if this is ultimately what needs to happen.

An ideal mentoring team[1] should consist of individuals who can serve as your traditional mentor, coach, connector, and sponsor. Some examples of individuals who may fulfill this purpose include:

- People senior to you;
- People at your level;
- People within your industry and field;
- People outside your industry and field;
- A community of practice (people who do what you do across a region or organization, e.g., physician moms);
- Emeritus faculty or those who have retired.

Elite athletes have a team of specialists who help them succeed—an athletic coach, a personal trainer, a nutritionist, a sports psychologist, etc. In the same way, mentors should help mentees create their team of specialists with unique expertise. Consider a mentoring team for someone interested in organizational systems—a primary mentor from their clinical specialty, someone with expertise in learning health systems, an implementation scientist, and a C-suite leader may be ideal.

By surrounding yourself with a team of mentors, you protect yourself from the negative side of a mentoring power dynamic and have an extra set of eyes to recognize the dysfunctional mentoring relationship, even if you are blinded to it.

Setting Project Timelines and Holding Mentors Accountable

If your mentor is a bottleneck, perhaps by not getting feedback to you in time or meeting with you at a regular cadence, manage up. Be clear about when and why you need something from them. Let them know that delays are harming your progress and that you need their support to be successful. It's helpful to also be crystal clear about what may happen if your mentor misses deadlines (e.g., "If I don't hear from you by the end of day Monday, I'll assume you don't have any objections to my submitting the paper"). If they repeatedly miss due dates, it may be time to think about getting a new mentor who has better time management or bandwidth. On the other hand, you may also be at a stage where your mentor doesn't feel like they need to hold your hand as much. If so, a conversation about becoming more independent and autonomous with your decision making can also be helpful in managing a bottleneck mentor.

Use Normative Pressure

While it should never be the intention to humiliate others, normative pressure can be powerful. Your mentor will likely be embarrassed knowing that their poor mentoring behaviors may become common knowledge among their peers. Of course, you must be prudent about how this is shared publicly. No one enjoys having their shortcomings paraded in public. A reasonable approach is to share your concerns with senior colleagues during performance reviews or other occasions where you have the opportunity to interact. Be tactful in how this happens—you don't want to run afoul of your mentor, especially if they don't fully appreciate how their delays are hurting your progress.

Knowing When and How to Walk Away

Sometimes, no matter how hard you try, the mentoring relationship is just not working out and doing you more harm than good. If that is the case, recognize it (see Table 10.1 for help identifying it), and be willing and ready to sever the mentoring relationship. This is by no means a simple task, but it's far better to leave than to let a poorly matched mentorship continue. This requires some carefully thought-out planning and guidance from people who know you and your delicate situation.

Planning Your Exit

Okay, you've made the decision to end the mentoring relationships. While you may wish to have a dramatic exit filled with fireworks and flare, we would advise against burning bridges. One size rarely fits all; for these challenging—and oftentimes emotionally charged—situations, understanding some effective solutions can help you manage matters with aplomb.

1. **Have a backup plan:** Think things through and play out several scenarios. Make sure you have a plan for what will happen next in those situations. Ensure you have a place to go to start a new mentoring

relationship before ending the current one. You will need to control the narrative before this happens.

2. **Make a decision and commit to it:** Once you have made the decision to move on, commit to the decision and follow through, even if the original mentor promises to change. If you've gotten to this point, you have already had some heart-to-heart conversations, and the tormentor mentor has not changed their behavior. Therefore, there is no reason to believe they will do so now. Move forward, commit.

3. **Maintain professionalism and avoid burning bridges:** Even though you are leaving, you want the relationship to end on the best terms possible. Remember, you initially chose this mentor for a reason—perhaps it was their success in the field, their expertise, network, or their ability to successfully mentor others. This continues to be the case. What has changed is that you have realized that the relationship is no longer conducive to your success as you believed it would be. But you don't want this mentor to become an enemy or someone who will prevent future success.

Handling a Mentoring Exit Professionally

Other than your immediate sense of gratification, it serves you no purpose to hurl accusations or personal attacks. In fact, it might work against you, as some may think you appear unhinged and less connected to the complexities of various issues. Provided the mentor has not done anything egregious and crossed any red lines (e.g., sexual harassment or racial discrimination, scientific misconduct, criminal abuse), airing out your professional laundry through public battles between an established mentor and a relatively unknown mentee usually doesn't end well. If those issues are at the root cause, then it is paramount that you take the appropriate steps within your organization's policies. Do not try to deal with them alone—elevate as appropriate and follow established norms for managing these problems. In the absence of egregious issues, aim for an amicable and professional separation whenever possible. See Table 10.2 for sample scripts to exit a mentoring relationship—use these scripts as models to end a mentoring relationship professionally and respectfully while maintaining positive connections in your field.

Ending a mentoring relationship is a natural part of career growth. With the right approach, you can transition gracefully while preserving valuable professional relationships.

TABLE 10.2 Professionally Ending a Mentoring Relationship

Ending on a Positive Note: Goals Achieved

Email	*e.g., A medical resident upon completing a rotation under a senior attending and is now moving into a fellowship requiring different expertise.*
Subject: Thank You for Your Mentorship Dear Dr. [Mentor's Last Name],	

I want to express my gratitude for your mentorship over the past [timeframe]. Your guidance has been invaluable in shaping my growth in [specific area, e.g., surgical training, medical research], and I truly appreciate the time and expertise you've shared.

As I transition into the next stage of my career, I feel it's the right time to seek additional mentorship to align with my evolving goals. I would love to stay in touch and continue learning from you in different capacities. Thank you again for everything.

Best regards,

[Your Name]

In-person Conversation

Dr. [Mentor's Last Name], I want to take a moment to thank you for your support over the past [timeframe]. Your mentorship has been incredibly valuable in my professional development. Now that I've reached a new phase in my career, I feel it's the right time to transition to different mentorship opportunities. I'd love to keep in touch, and I truly appreciate all that I've learned from you.

Transitioning to a Different Type of Mentor

Email	*e.g., A researcher in internal medicine who now wants to specialize in global health policy and needs a mentor in that field.*
Subject: Shifting My Mentorship Focus Dear Dr. [Mentor's Last Name],	

I want to sincerely thank you for the guidance and support you have provided. Your insights have been instrumental in my growth. As I focus more on [new goal, e.g., clinical specialization, academic leadership], I've realized I need mentorship that aligns more directly with this path.

I appreciate everything you've taught me and would love to stay in touch as I continue this journey. Thank you again for your support.

Best,

[Your Name]

(Continued)

TABLE 10.2 (Continued)

In-person Conversation

> Dr. [Mentor's Last Name], I've been reflecting on my professional goals and have realized that I now need mentorship in a slightly different direction. I truly appreciate everything you've taught me, and I want to make sure I continue growing in a way that aligns with my evolving career focus. I would love to stay connected and hope to continue learning from you in other ways.

Mentor is Unavailable or Too Busy

Email	*e.g., A junior faculty member who rarely gets time with their mentor (who is often traveling for global medical initiatives).*
Subject: Thank You for Your Support Dear Dr. [Mentor's Last Name],	

I truly appreciate the mentorship you have provided over the past [timeframe]. I understand how demanding your schedule is, and I know it can be challenging to find time for regular check-ins. To ensure I continue progressing, I've decided to seek additional mentorship with someone who has more availability for ongoing discussions.

I want to thank you for everything I have learned from you and hope we can remain in touch.

Warm regards,

[Your Name]

In-person Conversation

> Dr. [Mentor's Last Name], I completely understand how busy your schedule is, and I truly appreciate the time you've spent mentoring me. Given the demands of my current role, I realize I need more regular guidance to stay on track. I've decided to find additional mentorship to complement the foundation you've given me. I'm very grateful for your support and hope we can stay in touch.

Mentor's Approach No Longer Works for You

Email	*e.g., A surgical resident who realizes their mentor is more hands-off than they need for their next phase of training.*
Subject: Transitioning My Mentorship Relationship Dear Dr. [Mentor's Last Name],	

I want to express my appreciation for the guidance you've provided. Your mentorship has been instrumental in my career development. As I evaluate my next steps, I've realized I would benefit from a mentorship style that better aligns with my current needs.

This is a natural part of growth, and I sincerely value the time and effort you've invested in me. I look forward to staying in touch and continuing to learn from your expertise.

Best regards,

[Your Name]

(Continued)

TABLE 10.2 (Continued)

In-person Conversation

"Dr. [Mentor's Last Name], I truly appreciate your support and mentorship. As I continue to develop in my field, I've realized that my needs are shifting, and I would benefit from a different kind of mentorship at this stage. I want to thank you for all the time and insight you've given me, and I hope we can remain connected professionally."

Diplomatically Ending a Toxic Mentorship	
Email Subject: Moving Forward in My Mentorship Journey Dear Dr. [Mentor's Last Name],	*e.g., A research fellow whose mentor has repeatedly taken credit for their work or dismissed their contributions.*

I want to express my gratitude for the time and effort you have invested in my development. After reflecting on my professional needs, I've decided to transition to a mentorship that is a better fit for my current goals.

I appreciate the opportunities I have had to learn from you, and I hope we can part on good terms. Thank you again for your time and guidance.

Best,

[Your Name]

In-person Conversation

Dr. [Mentor's Last Name], I want to thank you for your time and the insights you've shared with me. After some reflection, I feel that I need to take a different direction with my mentorship to better align with my career goals. I appreciate everything I've learned from you, and I hope we can remain connected professionally.

Summary

As a mentee, staying attuned to your professional conduct and commitments is crucial. Ensure you deliver on promises and maintain a strong work ethic. But of equal importance is awareness of your mentor's behavior. Allowing a mentor to exploit or neglect their role can jeopardize your career. Be aware of the signs of mentorship malpractice, and be ready to speak up when you see them. If needed, know that you can exit the relationship at any time, and aim to do so amicably.

Hopefully, if you've chosen mentors whom you respect and admire, and you've had a positive mentoring experience full of growth and guidance, you may come to a point where it's simply time to move on. Your mentorship needs will evolve as your career goals shift, and needing new mentors with different experience and expertise is not surprising. Thank those who have spent time on you, and consider how you might pass along the knowledge and wisdom you've gleaned to the next generation of mentees.

Take-Home Points

- Learn to identify and address "red flag" behaviors that a mentor might exhibit. If you spot them, don't let them fester; address them immediately.
- Having a team of mentors creates a safety net for mentees by offering multiple perspectives and shared responsibilities, as well as providing advocates in case one relationship goes awry.
- It's better to end a bad mentoring relationship (even if doing so is uncomfortable!) than to risk the impact it will have on your career.

CHAPTER

11

Menteeship for Clinicians and Non-Researchers

When trying to find my way as an early career academic hospitalist, I knew I'd need help . . . and a lot of it. I needed a capital "M" mentor if I was going to survive, particularly given I was in a purely clinical appointment. As someone who prides themselves on their strong work ethic, self-sufficiency, and autonomy, I found this prospect frustrating and a bit defeating. I was intimidated by having to find that one perfect person whose interests aligned exactly with mine, and then trying to emulate their path to success. No autonomy, no individuality, no creativity.

However, something clicked, and I shifted my perspective. I didn't need to find "the one"; I could strategize to better leverage the academic community I worked with every day—the à la carte option! By pairing my individual interests or needs with multiple colleagues who had a distinct expertise in those areas, I realized I could get the best of both worlds. I could still carve my own path, but by learning from many rather than from one, I gained multiple perspectives, avoided overburdening a single mentor, and rapidly expanded my network. I didn't know it at the time, but this approach supercharged the trajectory of my academic learning and productivity, which was critical in the early stage of my career.

—**RJ Schildhouse, MD, University of Michigan Medical School**

In Chapter 7, we shared considerations for choosing a mentor. In the world of research, identifying a mentor can be relatively straightforward—your primary mentor is typically a senior, well-established investigator in your field of enquiry. Their role is clear and well-defined—helping with papers, grants, career advice—with structured expectations for mentorship. Success is defined by hitting milestones X, Y, and Z, and the primary mentor along with your mentorship team helps you achieve those milestones.

However, for physicians who spend most of their time in clinical education and patient care, mentorship is less clear-cut. Ditto for other non-research healthcare professionals, including advanced practice professionals, nurses, physical therapists, social workers, clinical pharmacists, psychologists, and other healthcare personnel. Who gets the "mentor" label can be a bit of an enigma. In a hospital or clinical setting, you work with different physicians, senior healthcare workers, and administrators on every shift. Is your mentor your residency director, your supervisor, your administrative boss, or an attending physician you admire? Perhaps it is the senior nurse who teaches you the unspoken rules of patient care. Or the administrator who is uber efficient and effective at managing direct and lateral reports.

The truth is, in healthcare, mentorship is often self-directed. With no designated mentor in most domains, the responsibility of cultivating meaningful mentorship often falls on the mentee. For this to work, you need to be intentional in your search for mentors. We'll explore how clinicians and non-research healthcare professionals can navigate this ambiguity, proactively seek mentorship, and build relationships that foster professional growth.

Assessing Your Mentorship Needs

As briefly mentioned in Chapter 7 and more extensively in Chapter 8, when searching for a mentor, consider where you need the most help and what gaps you wish to fill.[1] These will likely vary based on the stage of your career. For example, as a budding resident, your focus may be on how to be more prepared for rounds or presentations. Your senior residents are therefore likely the best source for mentorship as they too have had to face this task and surmount it to move forward. In contrast, when you are a junior faculty, your focus may be on honing your craft—whether that's improving your patient experience scores or learning how to develop a practice niche. Ask yourself what skills do you want to learn, where do you want to grow and develop further, and what are some short- and long-term goals? Examples of such goals may be getting into a fellowship, developing better work–life balance, learning leadership skills, or finding a job.

Box 11.1 offers some reflection questions to get you thinking about what you'd like a mentor's help with. Use this self-assessment tool to clarify career goals, identify skill gaps, and identify what you need from a mentor. Answer each question honestly to better understand the type of mentorship that will benefit you most.

Box 11.1 Assessing Your Mentorship Needs

1. **Career Goals**

   - What are your short-term career goals (next 1–3 years)?
   - What are your long-term career aspirations (5+ years)?
   - Do you want to specialize in a particular field or transition into a leadership role?
   - Are you considering a non-clinical path, such as hospital administration, medical education, or healthcare policy?
   - What challenges or barriers do you currently face in achieving these goals?
   - Who are some of the exemplars you see yourself becoming?

2. **Skill Gaps and Development Areas**

   - What clinical skills or areas of focus do you need to learn or improve to feel more confident in your role?
   - Are there administrative, leadership, or communication skills you need to develop?
   - If your goal is to be an educator, are there specific areas you would like to focus on, and how can you find your niche?
   - Do you struggle with work–life balance, time management, or stress management? Where are the areas for greatest growth for you?
   - Do you know how to manage people, space, and money?
   - Have you received feedback (formal or informal) about areas where you could improve?
   - Are you looking for mentorship to help with difficult conversations, conflict management, or negotiations?

3. **Ideal Mentor Characteristics**

   - What qualities do you value in a mentor (e.g., patience, accessibility, leadership experience, technical expertise)?

- Do you prefer a mentor who gives direct feedback or someone who takes a more supportive and guiding approach?
- Would you benefit more from a mentor within your organization or someone from an external professional network?
- Have you known or worked with individuals whom you respect or admire and under whom you would like to grow?
- Do you prefer structured mentorship (e.g., scheduled meetings) or informal check-ins?

4. **Finding the Right Mentor**

- Do you already have someone in mind who could be a mentor? If so, what about them makes them a good fit? Have they mentored others? Do you know any of their current or prior mentees?
- Have you observed someone in your workplace whose career path or leadership style you respect and admire?
- Are there professional organizations, societies, or institutional mentorship programs you could explore?

5. **Next Steps**

- What is one action you can take this month to seek mentorship?
- How will you reach out to a potential mentor (e.g., email, informal conversation, setting up a meeting)?
- What specific questions or topics would you like to discuss with a mentor in your first meeting?
- How can you plan your pitch to ask them to serve as a mentor, and what is it that you bring to the mentoring relationship that will help attract them to you?

Action plan: Based on your answers, write down three key takeaways about what you need in a mentor and one concrete step you will take to start your mentorship journey.

Identifying the Right Mentor in a Non-Research Context

Once you have a clearer indication of what you need and what you're seeking, you need to start your search in the right places. It's not about casting a wide net but rather casting your net in the right waters.

Within Your Department or Organization

Your ideal mentor, who can guide you, might be right under your nose. Look within your division, department, and organization to see who has the skills, mindset, and values you are seeking. Look people up on your organization's web pages. Run a PubMed search to see if they've done work in areas in which you are interested. Perhaps shadow them for a clinic or attend a seminar they are presenting. Going to Grand Rounds in your department is also a nice way to identify mentors. If the topic sounds interesting and the speaker seems engaging, you have someone to follow up with. Similarly, don't limit yourself to just your departmental seminars—attend talks in other departments. Institution-wide symposia and faculty development talks are all great ways to meet new people and learn about their work and see them in action. If you like what you see, introduce yourself after their talk and chat with them. After the event, follow up with an email—reintroduce yourself, explain what you liked about the talk and why you want to talk to them as a next step and for how long. Each of us has received emails such as this after talks we've given. A recent one went as follows:

Dear Dr. Chopra,

Thank you for visiting our organization and for your seminar focused on how to develop guidance for vascular device use in patients with cancer. The way you've approached a seemingly mundane topic with rigor and with an aim to improve clinical practice across specialties is inspiring and something I wish to emulate in my career.

As we discussed briefly after your presentation, I am a nurse working on ways to improve how nurses assess the venous circulation in an effort to prevent harm from peripheral IV insertion. My aim is to develop a curriculum that is pragmatic, can be applied to nurses as they develop their clinical skills, and has milestones and metrics for success. Like your work, I believe the creation of such courses meets an unfilled need and can help improve patient safety.

If you would be willing, I would appreciate 30 minutes of your time to meet and share my ideas with you. Your feedback would help me further develop and refine my ideas. I would be most grateful for your support.

Outside Your Department or Organization

The first myth worth busting is that your mentor doesn't have to be the person directly supervising you—it could be someone from another department, a senior administrator, or even a peer (friendtor)[2] with more experience in a particular area. Look both within and outside your department, organization, and industry. You may be a neurologist, but that doesn't mean everyone who mentors you should be a neurologist, and certainly not confined to the neurology department at your organization. Perhaps a gastroenterologist or basic scientist in industry has found a solution to the problem you are facing.

Branch out. Join various groups on social media, WhatsApp, or Slack, and follow individuals whom you admire. The idea is if you follow them, you will learn about opportunities where you can join in, learn, and potentially meet new mentors. The University of Colorado and University of Michigan jointly sponsor a Mentorship Academy, which is open to all healthcare workers, and they rotate the location of the symposium between the two universities.[3] For one day, people can hear talks and panels from mentoring experts from all over the United States (and a few from outside its borders). They learn how to approach people, how to mentor and be mentored effectively, and how to develop teams; hear case studies; etc. Following leaders in mentorship on social media is one way you can learn of such events.

Assigned Mentors

Some organizations have formal mentoring programs, which you should investigate as well. For example, the Department of Medicine at the University of Colorado has programs focused on Launch (junior faculty in their first few years) and Boost (mid-career/senior faculty) teams.[4] These programs aim to create a group of mentors around individuals at key steps of their development. While research has shown that assigned mentors may be less fruitful than organically found ones,[5,6] when you are starting out, it is helpful to have at least one person you can talk to. The entire purpose of some of these programs is to better refine your career direction, orient you to the resources available on campus, and position you to find your niche and mentoring needs. As you become more comfortable, you can further expand and explore your mentoring circle.

Assigned mentors are helpful to those who may not naturally tend to reach out to others for help. Statistically, women, those who are reserved, and people from certain cultures may not make the first move, so assigned mentors solve that problem.[7] They are also a nice way to create a culture of mentorship. Departments and programs that offer these types of initiatives say a lot about their priorities and how they value growth of people.

Professional Societies

Professional societies can also be great resources for expanding your mentorship circle. Being part of these societies through committee work or through attending national meetings introduces you to how other organizations work. They provide ways to connect with people outside your organization who may be doing work similar to yours or in spaces where you have interest. Being part of these organizations can help expand your network, such that when you need to establish your national presence, you have a circle you can turn to. When the time comes, the people you connect with and continue to keep in contact with might write you letters of recommendation for your academic promotion. Your mentor within a professional society can also recommend you for talks, panels, and other opportunities within the society: all things that will help you learn and grow and make a strong case for your promotion.

The goal is to identify people who have the experience and insight you need and then work to build a relationship with them. Finding the right mentor isn't always straightforward, but by being proactive, seeking out the right qualities, and thinking beyond traditional hierarchies and your own organization, you can create a network of mentors who will help guide your career in ways you never expected.

See Table 11.1 for proactive ideas of where to look for a mentor, and how to approach them (including scripts). The critical step is initiating and the follow-up. We are all flooded with emails, and most don't get read. You may need to send out more than one email to ensure yours percolates to the top and gets seen. After your meeting, be sure to follow up with the 24/7/30 format.[8] Within 24 hours after you meet someone, reach out with an email. Seven days later, follow up again, often circling back to something that was discussed, or sharing a related resource such as an article or podcast interview that discusses the exact thing you were talking about. Thirty days later, you reach out again and share how you applied the lessons from the conversation, what worked, and what didn't. This type of cadence and persistence helps show your commitment to the relationship.

TABLE 11.1 Six Proactive Strategies for Seeking Mentorship

Where to Seek	How to Approach	Example Script
Within Your Department	Ask a senior colleague for a 20-minute meeting to discuss strategies for managing complex cases.	"Dr. [Name], I've been working on improving my efficiency in managing multiple patients on rounds. Would you be open to a 20-minute conversation to share how you approach it?"
Professional Societies and Conferences	Follow up with a speaker after a conference session and ask for a quick discussion on their career path in a specific field.	"I really enjoyed your talk at [conference/event], especially your points on physician leadership. I'm exploring similar career paths and find myself stuck identifying opportunities beyond the obvious—would you have 20 minutes to share how you got started?"
Hospital Leadership and Administration	Request a 20-minute conversation with a department chair or hospital leader to learn about leadership pathways within your organization.	"I'm considering stepping into a leadership role of division chief in my department but want to understand the challenges involved. Could we schedule a 20-minute chat about your experience making that transition?"
Interdisciplinary Teams	Reach out to an experienced nurse, therapist, or pharmacist for a conversation about improving collaboration between teams.	"It's no secret that effective teamwork between physicians and nurses makes a big difference in patient outcomes. I'd love to hear your perspective on improving collaboration—would you be open to a 20-minute conversation so that we can brainstorm?"
Alumni Networks	Contact an alum from your medical school/residency program for a virtual coffee chat about career transitions.	"We both trained at [institution], and I'm at a career crossroads similar to one you've navigated. Would you be open to a 20-minute virtual coffee chat to discuss how you approached your decision to leave academic medicine for private practice?"
Online Communities and Social Media	Engage in a professional discussion on social media, Slack, or WhatsApp, then ask for a short call to exchange insights.	"I appreciated your recent LinkedIn post on preventing burnout in healthcare. I'm working on improving this for the members of my team and would love to hear what's worked for you and what hasn't. Would you be open to a quick 20-minute chat?"

Mentorship as a Path to Skill Development

Joe was an expert clinician and educator. He trained thousands of medical students in his 20 years at the organization where he worked. He wanted a new challenge and was looking into how he might join the organization's leadership in an educational leadership capacity. He reached out to his division chief, who was his mentor for years, and asked for recommendations as to others who had similar leadership roles. He explained his goal was to determine what skills he needed versus what skills he currently had. With the delta clear to him, he proposed to develop a mentorship team that could help him fill that gap. In Joe's case, he had all the right instructional skills. What he needed to learn was how to manage people and budgets and develop curricula that could be aligned with these aspects. See Table 11.2 for a list of skills a mentor might be able to help you with.

Mentorship isn't just about career advice—it's a useful tool to develop new skills that will define your success in healthcare and help you stand out. Perhaps you are years post-residency or about to take on a new leadership role, as Joe wanted to do. The truth is that there are always new skills to learn, new paths to navigate, and new opportunities to explore. Formal classroom instruction might not be appropriate or relevant to many of these aspects. So how will you learn these skills? Whether you're working at a bedside, in the operating room, managing a unit, or transitioning into a leadership role, the right mentorship can teach you the necessary skills and accelerate your growth in ways that formal training alone cannot.

Sometimes, decisions need to be made in the moment, and that is nearly impossible to teach via a textbook. For example, take clinical decision making. No matter how many textbooks you've read or question banks you've answered, nothing really prepares you for the decisions you might need to make in a difficult case or when running a code. Observing an experienced healthcare provider navigate high-pressure situations, prioritize care, and communicate empathetically with patients and families is invaluable. In these settings, a mentor doesn't just teach you protocols—they show you how to think critically during stressful situations, how to trust your instincts, and how to handle the inevitable emotional weight of the job. Not all emergencies are created equal, and mentors can help you recognize and differentiate between time-bound and non-time-bound emergency decisions.[9]

Mentorship isn't just for honing your clinical expertise. If you have aspirations beyond direct patient care, a mentor can help you develop the leadership and management skills needed to take on more responsibility. They

TABLE 11.2 Skills to Develop with a Mentor Based on Career Stage

Career Stage	Skills (Example)
Early	Clinical decision making (Triaging cases in the emergency department)
	Patient communication (Delivering difficult diagnoses with empathy)
	Time management (Balancing patient load during residency)
	Interdisciplinary collaboration (Working with nurses and therapists through post-operative care)
	Work–life balance (Managing shift work and personal well-being)
Middle	Leadership and management (Supervising a hospital unit or clinic)
	Advanced clinical skills (Mastering robot-assisted surgery)
	Conflict resolution (Handling disputes between physicians and nursing staff)
	Navigating hospital politics (Advocating for departmental resources)
	Career advancement (Transitioning from clinical work to hospital administration)
Senior	Strategic decision making (Shaping hospital policies related to patient care)
	Mentoring others (Guiding junior physicians and residents)
	Public speaking and advocacy (Representing a medical institution at conferences)
	Change management (Implementing a new electronic health record system)
	Legacy and succession planning (Preparing the next generation of departmental leaders)

can recommend specific skills that would be useful, teach you how to navigate institutional politics, inform you of the hidden curriculum—those rules you are supposed to know but are never codified—find out which meetings you must go to and which are worth skipping, whom to trust and whom to watch out for, and so much more. Moving from clinician to leader requires an entirely different skillset—one where, perhaps for the first time, you will need to be responsible for people, time, and space.

You will need to learn budgeting, conflict resolution, strategic decision making, politics, navigating institutional norms and managing above and below you—skills that aren't part of any formal school curriculum (even for many MBA programs). A mentor who has been down this road before you can help you anticipate challenges, build confidence, avoid common pitfalls, and develop a team of allies.

Healthcare is a multidisciplinary sport, yet working effectively across disciplines doesn't come naturally to many. In fact, much of healthcare is based on individual success in terms of propelling you forward. But the truth is that we never do it alone, and there is never just one way to be successful. Physicians, nurses, allied health professionals, and administrators all have different needs, pressures, perspectives, priorities, and ways of communicating. Even within the same type of healthcare provider, these may vary. A good mentor can teach you how to bridge that divide and get everyone working together as in a choreographed dance.

At every stage of your career, mentorship isn't just about career advice—it's about developing the skills that will allow you to thrive in an ever-evolving healthcare landscape. The key is recognizing what you need and seeking out the right mentors to help you get there.

Overcoming Common Challenges in Non-Research Mentorship

When You Don't Control Your Time

For those who work in the clinical space, their time is not their own. You can't cancel a case, close the OR, or send patients home today because you need a meeting with your mentor. Carving out time for mentorship can be a real test of your scheduling skills. You may not have time for a full one-hour meeting, so make the most of brief interactions. Instead of covering multiple topics, focus on one or two and save smaller issues for email. Take advantage of making time-in-time. Prepare to have meetings when you travel, in the hallway in the hospital, in the breakroom, or when on call together. Have a list on your phone of topics you'd like to discuss when you see your mentor. Some challenges can be solved with a quick hallway conversation or a coffee together while on call. Make the most of the time you have with your mentor.

Navigating Clinical Hierarchies

Clinical settings are steeped in hierarchies and traditions, which can make the mentorship complex, *if* you are unclear of where you fit within this structural paradigm. Respecting everyone you work with—at every level and role—and treating them with dignity is a baseline requirement, which should be obvious (but, sadly, people forget). No matter how smart or skilled you are, how you engage with colleagues, senior leaders, attendings, administrators, and interdisciplinary teams can either stifle or grow your career. The key is learning how to seek guidance and mentorship while respecting the chain of command, ensuring that mentorship enhances rather than disrupts workplace dynamics.

Managing Multiple Mentors

As we discussed in Chapter 1, having a team of mentors is essential to ensuring you are tapping into multiple skills, perspectives, and networks. It is not uncommon to have multiple mentors: one for clinical expertise, another for research, and yet another for leadership development and navigating hospital politics. We fully endorse this approach. To effectively leverage these relationships, you need to have clarity, knowing when and for what to approach each mentor.

If you are consistently going for "second opinions" until you get the one you agree with, that is a poor utilization of your mentors' limited time and frankly will annoy them if you make this a habit.

Summary

For healthcare workers who spend most of their time in education and clinical care, as opposed to research, mentorship may be less clear-cut. In the hospital setting, you work with many knowledgeable and skilled people, but only a select few can be a part of your mentoring team. This is why it's important to assess your mentoring needs. Identify the skills you must gain, your career goals, those who possess the qualities you value in a mentor, and what action you can take to move forward. While these individuals may be in your department or organization, branch out and consider those at other organizations or society meetings. Perhaps your division has a formal mentoring program. Consider all options to form a well-rounded, carefully crafted team of mentors. This team is designed to support you beyond just career advice—they help you develop all the necessary skills to thrive in healthcare.

Take-Home Points

- Know your mentorship needs before asking a new mentor to meet with you. Identify what skills or knowledge you have gaps in, what goals you have, and who embodies an ideal mentor.
- Your next mentor might be someone you share a department with, or maybe not. Look beyond your organization to see what individuals inspire you and you desire to learn from. Social media or society meetings can be great for connecting people.
- A team of mentors is the best approach for well-rounded mentorship. Different perspectives, experience, and expertise benefits you—don't stick to one individual out of fear of offending!

III

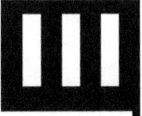

Working Together

12

Mentoring across Generations: Find Your Common Ground

In the 1990s, when the internet first took the world by storm, Jack Welch, the former CEO of General Electric, recognized this was an emerging technology, and his senior executives, who were generally older, needed to understand this new market. Welch instructed his senior leaders to learn about the internet from the junior employees who were becoming digital natives, a practice now known as reverse mentoring.

The Welch example highlights how every person, of every generation, has different experiences and perspectives. Sometimes, we can look at these experiences through a new lens and gain new insights. Mentorship is an ideal tool to bridge generational gaps.

While age and generational influences don't—or shouldn't—matter in mentorship, we're human, so they do. While we inherently believe that guiding someone toward their best self should not be bound by time or cultural barriers, the reality is often quite different. Too often, good mentoring relationships lose momentum because of these generational differences.

Generational Awareness

These differences, simply put, are different roads to the same destination. But each path is shaped by a person's past experiences and upbringing, oftentimes making it difficult to recognize that there is another way to get there. Generational traits are widely studied[1,2] and written about,[3] yet it's almost impossible to fit people into rigid boxes, as not everyone fits the

DOI: 10.1201/9781003611233-15

generalizations. The goal, then, is not to stereotype—but rather to use these insights to improve mentorship through understanding what matters to a generation of people. By understanding these complexities, mentors and mentees can develop a mutual understanding. It reduces friction caused by different work styles (e.g., in person versus remote) and communication preferences (e.g., in-person meetings versus text). The more understanding that exists, the more the mentor and mentee can establish an effective relationship dynamic. See Table 12.1 for the five generations currently in the workplace, some generalized traits, the mediums they prefer to work in, and associated challenges as they relate to mentoring.[4]

There is a good chance your mentor or mentee will be from a different generation than you. Rather than focus on generational differences, focus on how they prefer to take in and process information.[5,6] Table 12.1 can give you some general insights into the matter, but it's best to ask the person directly. Consider asking questions on how they prefer to receive feedback, what their assumptions and hopes are for their career progression, their preferred style of communication, their work habits, etc. Before you get frustrated that the mentee or mentor doesn't understand or respect your unwritten rules of mentorship, have a conversation about it and avoid miscommunication.

There are countless exciting, productive, and enriching mentorship relationships that cross age and generational divides. The ideas about formal structure, communication, and timing might be vastly different from what you are accustomed to. To optimize the relationships, consider some of these tips. But please understand that we do not lump all individuals of any group and assume they want to be mentored in one specific way—we are speaking as epidemiologists and social scientists and making some generalizations with the hope of minimizing intergenerational misunderstandings.

Short and Targeted Interactions

The world has evolved at a rapid pace. What was new and exciting last year is expired today. It's easy to forget how much the ever changing world molds and defines those who grew up in it. Just three decades ago, the internet was not a central feature in most workplaces. Yet today our mentees and future workforce don't recognize a world without it. They are digital natives, and those who have entered the workforce in the last quarter of a century are used to having information at their fingertips at record speeds.

TABLE 12.1 Typical Generational Traits and Work Styles

Generation (Born)	Associated Traits	Work Style	Work Motivation	Mentorship Challenges
Traditionalist/Silent Generation (~1925~1945)	• Loyal • Disciplined • Respect authority	• Hierarchical • Structured • Formalized	• Job security • Recognition of hard work • Loyalty	• Rapid policy and procedure changes • Digital communication
Baby Boomer (~1946~1964)	• Competitive • Career-focused • Value experience	• Structured • Face-to-face interaction	• Job stability • Prestige and promotion • Respect for tenure	• Non-traditional mentoring arrangements
Gen X (~1965~1980)	• Adaptable • Independent • Question authority	• Flexible • Pragmatic • Work–life balance	• Autonomy • Efficiency • Direct communication	• May not seek mentorship • May resist structured feedback
Millennial (~1981~1996)	• Collaborative • Purpose-driven • Digital natives	• Informal • Team-oriented • Feedback-driven	• Purpose • Innovation • Meaning in work	• Prefer instant feedback • May challenge traditional structures
Gen Z (~1997~2012)	• Entrepreneurial • Socially conscious • Diverse	• Multitasking • Digital-first • Adaptive	• Personal growth • Career agility • Inclusivity	• Expecting rapid career growth • Impatience with progress

Millennials and Gen Zs in particular entered the workforce accustomed to a world of information at their fingertips via smartphones and other devices. This upbringing has conditioned them to crave instant, succinct, and direct communication via technologies such as texting and social media. These tools have shaped the last two generations of the workforce, transforming Millennials and Gen Zs into employees who thrive on accessibility and collaboration—something that simply wasn't possible when some mentors were embarking on their careers. This isn't a bad thing. Understanding their thought processes, just as they should strive to understand yours, can foster more effective mentoring relationships.

Millennials and Gen Zs are more likely to send a quick email or text or even drop in with a question while working on a project. Don't misunderstand their intentions—they're not trying to be disruptive. They've simply grown up in an environment where instant communication and collaboration are the norm. Waiting until next week's scheduled meeting doesn't align with the way they've been conditioned to work. Simply put, they need a different approach to mentorship.[7]

Micro-Mentoring

Frequent and short touchpoints can be an extremely efficient way to communicate and accomplish tasks. Instead of pushing back and insisting on rigid, formal meetings, embrace the two- to five-minute interaction in the hallway, by the coffee machine, or just before or after Grand Rounds or another seminar. These "micro-mentoring" sessions—frequent, brief, and highly focused meetings aimed at accomplishing specific tasks—enable your mentee to check in with you as needed. These can also be thought of as "constructive collisions" as they can enhance both mentoring and collaborative relationships. It is one of the reasons working remotely can be challenging, and why there is specific guidance on how to mentor in a remote environment.[8]

In today's day and age, filled with pings and dings from emails and text messages, we're acclimated to constant disruptions. If you really need some uninterrupted, focused time, discuss this with your mentee so they understand when it's acceptable to interrupt—and when they will have to wait. Ruth puts a "do not disturb" sign on her door when she's in deep, focused work or on Zoom calls and has instructed those around her that, when the sign is on the door, unless it's an emergency, she is not to be interrupted.

Beyond Hierarchy

The traditional form of mentoring, where the mentor is senior in experience and stature and plays a subordinate role is a foreign concept to today's mentees who were raised with open floor plans, flat hierarchy, and direct access to leadership via social media. That doesn't mean they lack respect for their superiors. Instead, today's mentees are more accustomed to being more transparent and to an open structure that enables them to communicate freely with everyone—from a new intern to the department chair, dean, or president of the hospital—without the need to follow traditional hierarchical channels.

This might sound horrifying to those who grew up in the era of starched white lab coats for rounds, instead of the Patagonia worn by today's young physicians. It's tempting to default to the position that the mentee may have no respect for authority or appreciation of a protocol for communicating with those in leadership. But this is not a helpful approach for your mentoring relationship.

Most likely the mentee is simply trying to be efficient. They may think that going through two people to approach the Chief Human Resources Officer or department chair is a waste of time, especially when they can quickly send an email directly to that person. After all, if they can get the information they need without troubling anyone else, why shouldn't they? Remember, they grew up in an age of email and LinkedIn where you can directly reach the leader of any organization. It's as natural to them as breathing.

These mentees often also believe that such acts show initiative. While this mentee might not be accustomed to strict hierarchies, the traditional structure may not be as open to change. Going directly to top leadership could be seen as inappropriate and may inadvertently harm the mentee's reputation. Teach your mentee how to navigate the hierarchy of your department and organization—what works, what doesn't, who is more or less approachable, how the culture works, and the rules of engagement. Healthcare—like the military—was built on hierarchies, and they are slow to change.

Purpose, Not Process

Today's mentees often prioritize purpose over process. They need to understand why they are doing things. The big picture is critical. They focus on making a meaningful impact—on their mentor, their team, and the world around them. The details become superfluous to the outcome. They are less interested in the details of how a mentor may think the task should be accomplished or the series of steps they should follow. Instead, they often believe that they are creative thinkers and nimble enough to figure things out on their own. Often, they are. It's not surprising if you remember that they are digital natives who figured out how to upload and download documents long before others and independently troubleshoot when the computer crashed. They often leverage the vast array of digital resources available to them, sometimes outperforming their mentor—and even teaching them something new in the process. Other times, they may need some scaffolding, even when they insist that they don't. It is the mentor's responsibility to discern when the mentee can independently handle something and when it is time to intervene, to help prevent poor judgment or critical mistakes that may compromise the mentee's career.

What motivates today's young mentees is whether the work they do will make a difference—whether it has purpose. When the work is aligned with their values, they are all in. Therefore, traditional metrics valued by previous generations—such as notoriety, wealth, accolades, or profession-specific benchmarks such as citation indexes—may hold less relevance for today's mentees. Instead, today's emerging mentees are asking themselves different questions: How will this make the world a better place? Is this interesting to me? Will it make me and others happy? Mentors can help the mentee visualize and articulate a larger picture and broader impact for the current work; they can help them understand how it might help humanity at large or see how a specific project may lead to contributions beyond traditional academic yardsticks. These ideals are attractive and motivating to today's incoming healthcare workforce. Simultaneously, the mentor must emphasize to the mentee the importance of professional metrics—citations, publications, and presentations at conferences do matter. These metrics will influence not only their career trajectory but also their ability to achieve their broader goals. The mentors who can do this balancing act and do it well are more likely to have positive relationships with young mentees than others. See Table 12.2 for mentoring tips for both mentor and mentee based on the generation of each.

TABLE 12.2 Cross-Generational Tips for Both Mentor and Mentee

Generation	For Mentors	For Mentees
Traditionalist/ Silent Generation	• Acknowledge mentee's experience and expertise • Use structured, formal mentoring approaches	• Respect mentor's structured approach • Be open to learning from mentor's deep experience
Baby Boomer	• Recognize mentee's contributions • Balance traditional and modern mentoring styles	• Acknowledge mentor's experience • Be patient with traditional mentoring methods
Gen X	• Respect mentee's independence • Offer flexible, clear, pragmatic guidance	• Communicate efficiently and directly • Appreciate mentor's balance of autonomy and mentorship
Millennial	• Emphasize purpose and impact • Provide regular feedback • Encourage collaboration	• Adapt to hierarchical structures • Understand the value of professional metrics
Gen Z	• Offer rapid feedback and growth opportunities • Embrace digital communication	• Be patient with career progression • Learn to navigate workplace hierarchy

Summary

Generational differences can introduce challenges to an effective mentoring relationship, but navigating such challenges is doable. Everyone has a unique background and preferences, and generation (or cohort) effects influence those preferences and differences. Though mentoring methods may differ from person to person, remember these are all different roads to the same destination. Most people are looking for similar things despite when they were born—they simply pursue them in a different manner, shaped by the environment in which they grew up.

We recommend trying to understand the preferences of those in other generations. If your mentor is a generation or two ahead of you, be open to learning from their experience, and be patient with traditional methods. If you find yourself mentoring someone a generation or two behind you—and may be struggling to comprehend their rapid, informal communication style—know that they value your feedback and collaboration and that their communication style reflects generational norms and not disrespect. Adopting a different approach can help you, as a mentor, grow.

While difficult, do your best to avoid assuming that different styles or learning strategies indicate a lack of patience, respect, or collaboration. Crossing generational lines can be enlightening, as both mentors and mentees aim for successful careers. Practicing and encouraging the timeless values of honesty, integrity, respect, and hard work still apply.

Take-Home Points

- Recognize and acknowledge generational differences that can pose challenges but be careful not to stereotype someone based on their age. Diverse experiences and preferences enrich mentorship. Overcome challenges by seeking to understand one another and your differences.
- Younger generations, such as Millennials and Gen Zs, value frequent, concise interactions over traditional long meetings. They often prioritize purpose over process. Effective mentoring therefore requires adapting to these communication styles, recognizing that approaches like direct communication with leaders stem from a desire for efficiency rather than disrespect.
- Today's mentees seek meaningful impact and may value alignment over conventional metrics. Mentors should help mentees visualize the broader impact of their work while emphasizing the importance of professional metrics for career progression. A successful mentorship balances purpose with guiding the mentee's progress using the necessary metrics.

13

Mentorship and Leadership: Where Paths Converge

Mentorship *requires* leadership. On the other hand, we *request* that leaders mentor.[1] Often, leadership is mistaken for mentorship, but it is important to appreciate that the responsibilities and skills differ. While the roles have overlapping traits, they are distinct entities. Longevity with a singular employer is dwindling, which means your leader—whether your division chief, department chair, or dean—will change. Consequently, your mentor, who is there for the long haul, may now be more critical than ever.

Research has shown that currently practicing physicians of all ages stayed with their first job out of residency for an average of six years.[2] Among physicians who have completed residency within the past six years, that average is down to less than two years. This lack of stability may be due to many reasons, including the decline in tenure-track positions[3] in academic medical centers. Between 1982 and 2022, the percentage of full-time physician faculty in tenure or tenure-track roles decreased from 59 to 18%. The basic sciences don't look that much better. Their tenure-track positions decreased from 78% to 64% during the same period.[4]

This is important, as your assigned leader may come and go, but your mentors will be in your life for years, even decades. In the past, people often stayed with a single employer for the long haul, even their entire career. It was common to hear faculty say that they trained at the very organization where they worked. Faculty frequently remained at the organizations where they trained. Today, however, there's a noticeable shift: healthcare professionals—including physicians, nurses, and other staff—are changing jobs more frequently and have much shorter tenures on faculty.

Often the two roles of mentor and leader are so intertwined that we can't distinguish where one ends and the other begins. The roles of mentor and leader naturally complement and reinforce each other. Effective mentors utilize core leadership skills such as communication, empathy, and strategic thinking.[5] Conversely, strong leaders lean on mentorship strategies, such as guiding, encouraging, developing, and nurturing talent.

Mentor–Leader Framework

To truly excel, mentorship and leadership should be seen as a continuum that develops both people and the organization, not distinct roles. There is a great deal of overlap with the responsibilities of a mentor and a leader. Within healthcare, effective mentors naturally exhibit leadership qualities, so it naturally becomes self-fulfilling and continuous. We developed the Mentor–Leader Framework to guide you. This framework has four quadrants that outline the core competencies seen in mentor–leaders. Figure 13.1 provides a visual to help you consider where you might fall within the four quadrants and where you need to grow.

1. **Trust:** Edelman, a leading communications and public relations firm, conducts an annual study they refer to as the Edelman Trust Barometer.[6] In over two decades, they've surveyed over two million people globally. The barometer revealed some truths. People have expectations of those they work with. They want to feel included, have a voice in decision making, and be in a culture that aligns with their values.

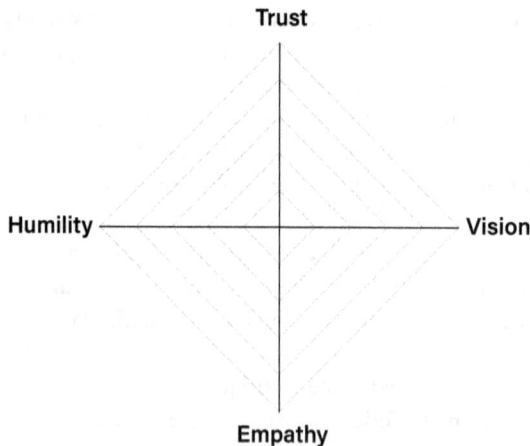

FIGURE 13.1 Four quadrants of the mentor–leader framework.

The 2022 Edelman report revealed that when the organization lives up to these expectations, employees trust them. And when employees' trust is secured, 83% of employees are committed to doing great work, 80% are loyal to the organization, and 82% advocate for the organization. Conversely, when trust is lacking, only 45% of employees are committed to doing great work, 36% have a sense of loyalty, and 35% will advocate for the organization.[7]

There is good news. Sometimes, small numbers can drive big results. In his book on trust, *To Be Honest*,[8] author Ron Carucci explains that if you "improve alignment between who you say you are and what you do by even 25%, you can increase employees' truth telling, just behavior, and purpose driven actions by 10%." This shows that it's not a zero-sum game. Incremental improvements can have a big impact. Never has this been more evident than with mentoring.

That's because an undisputed fact is that at the core of any mentoring relationship is trust. Effective mentors establish trust by demonstrating reliability, transparency, occasional vulnerability, and consistency. They ask for ideas and insights, align their work with their values, and help the mentee do the same. In leadership, trust is a necessary component for positive team dynamics; it encourages honest dialogue and loyalty and fosters a psychologically safe environment where individuals feel safe to innovate and grow.[9]

2. **Vision:** Sometimes, we are so deep inside the jar, we cannot read the label. Successful mentors clearly articulate a vision for their mentees' potential, encouraging them to see beyond immediate challenges. They show them that they believe in their potential and where that can lead. They plant seeds of inspiration and show them the path.

    In the same vein, strong leaders effectively communicate an inspiring vision that motivates and unites teams toward shared goals. When there are shared goals that everyone can rally around, implementation becomes so much more coordinated and effective. Team members see themselves not as individual contributors but as part of a collective. They understand that if they don't do their part, it will impact others.

3. **Empathy:** One of the differentiators between a mentor and a coach is that the mentor previously traveled the path the mentee is on, while a coach may not have the same experience or expertise. The shared journey, albeit at different time periods, allows mentors to leverage empathy in order to deeply understand their mentees' perspectives and experiences, creating a shared understanding. They are able to put themselves in the mentee's shoes, as they've walked in them. Whether a complicated clinical

case, failed experiments, rejected manuscripts, or poor scores on grants, the mentor has been there and knows how it feels. They fully understand the struggle when things go wrong and the elation when things work out.

Empathy in leadership is not too dissimilar as it shows that you genuinely care about those you lead. It creates a pivotal supportive environment, which is so necessary and often overlooked in healthcare. Empathy strengthens interpersonal relationships by showing every member of the healthcare team that their lived experiences, feelings, and perspectives are necessary and valued. It fosters stronger interpersonal relationships, encourages emotional intelligence among the team members, and promotes inclusive, compassionate decision making.

4. **Humility:** In his book, *The Purpose Driven Life*, Rick Warren aptly states, "Humility is not thinking less of yourself, it's thinking of yourself less."[10] It is this exact thinking that drives successful mentors. Exceptional mentors recognize their own limits, continuously engage in self-reflection, and remain open to learning alongside their mentees. They measure their success not simply by their own accomplishments, but by those of their mentees.

Conversely, leaders who embrace humility encourage an organizational culture of lifelong learning, openness, and continuous improvement. Satya Nadella, the CEO of Microsoft, transformed his company's culture by telling every employee to "Stay humble, stay hungry, and exhibit a growth mindset." He wanted his employees to have a "learn-it-all" instead of a "know-it-all" attitude.

These concepts align well with the field of "positive leadership." For example, in his book *Positive Energizing Leadership*, Kim Cameron from the University of Michigan—one of the field's pioneers—provides ample evidence that simple virtuous acts by the leader generate positive relational energy, which serves to attract and inspire high-quality employees.[11] What are these virtuous behaviors? Compassion, generosity, gratitude, trustworthiness, forgiveness, and kindness. In a word: Love.[12] Positive energizing mentors likely exhibit similar behaviors.

Adult Learning: The Secret to Stronger Leadership

Successful mentorship is not left to chance. It's intentional, reflective, and, knowingly or not, grounded in adult learning principles. Many successful mentors intuitively use adult learning strategies. They naturally encourage and push their mentees to reflect, ask questions, take ownership of their learning, and go down a rabbit hole when something is of unique interest to them; this is also known as self-directed learning, experiential learning, and transformative learning.

Adult learning, academically referred to as andragogy, beautifully intersects with leadership, primarily the following three learning theories.

Self-Directed Learning

In this case, mentees take ownership of their learning. Self-directed learning can be a goal, a process, or an attribute. You might recognize this in a mentee who independently researches evidence-based practices, then shares the information with their mentor, or in a junior attending who recognizes the potential of virtual reality in healthcare and signs up for a specialized training program or attends a conference on the topic.

This aligns with the self-leadership skills described by Malcolm Knowles, the grandfather of andragogy, in his early work.[13] Knowles underscores that those who are self-directed will take the initiative to diagnose and go after their needs. They set goals, evaluate outcomes, reflect, and strive for autonomy and lifelong learning. The mentor can encourage the self-directed learning by making them feel at ease, supporting them, helping them articulate their learning needs, involving them in the planning of their own career and learning path, making learning a mutual responsibility, and using methods that draw on the mentee's prior knowledge.

Experiential Learning

The age-old saying see one, do one, teach one is based on experiential learning. The entirety of clinical clerkships are too. We learn by rolling up our sleeves and doing the work. The learning is directly linked to an encounter with what is being done, instead of just thinking about it. The learning occurs because of the direct participation in the event. David Kolb and others underscore that adults take in and process information differently, but the experiential learning is an anchor among all of them.[14] The experience forms new knowledge, and careful reflection of that experience develops new understandings that can then lead a mentee to take action, based on the new insights.

This can be seen in simulation labs, where after each simulation, the team members discuss and then reflect on their decision, actions, and communication. This develops and enhances their clinical judgment, collaboration, and communication skills.

Transformative Learning

Jack Mezirow's theory of transformative learning explains that adults often experience an "aha moment"—a pivotal event that causes them to question their long-held assumptions.[15] This realization encourages deep reflection, opening their minds to new possibilities and ultimately inspiring them to take action in new and meaningful ways. At the core of this process is the transformative learning experience itself—the event or insight that sparks profound change.

Imagine a physician who is experiencing burnout, after working nonstop for years. After a series of conversations with her mentor, the mentee realizes that her assumptions about productivity and work–life balance are off-kilter. She starts to develop boundaries and becomes an advocate for physician wellness initiatives in the hospital.

Another example might be a nurse manager who is facing significant turnover in his department. After a conversation with his mentor, he recognizes that his traditional hierarchical leadership approach is ineffective, and his direct communication is coming off as abrasive. He gives this some thought and works to develop a new leadership approach that is collaborative and significantly improves employee satisfaction and engagement.

Applying Adult Learning Principles in Healthcare Mentoring Relationships

There are many ways to integrate mentoring based on adult learning strategies. Use the following bullets as a guide to ensure that your mentorship aligns with adult learning principles, enhancing your mentees' growth as healthcare leaders.

Self-Directed Learning

- Encourage mentees (e.g., medical trainees, nurses, healthcare administrators) to establish clear personal goals, such as developing new clinical competencies, procedural skills, or leadership skills.
- Support mentees in independently identifying educational resources (journals, conferences, courses, certifications) relevant to their specialized interests or career path, and show them how best to use these resources for their growth.
- Guide mentees in creating personalized professional development plans, such as pursuing a fellowship or advanced training or a leadership role within their clinical department or specialty.

Experiential Learning

- Provide mentees opportunities for hands-on experiences, such as presenting at a team meeting, Grand Rounds, starting a difficult case, or writing the first draft of a manuscript.

- Facilitate structured reflection sessions after clinical experiences, critical incidents, patient safety incidents, or challenging patient interactions to highlight key learning points and become comfortable with talking through challenging issues.
- Create a supportive space for mentees to openly discuss successful clinical outcomes, challenges during a case, and areas for improvement.

Transformative Learning

- Prompt mentees to critically evaluate assumptions, such as patient care practices, team communication styles, or approaches to work–life balance.
- Encourage mentees to reflect deeply after significant events (patient loss, medical errors, data contamination, or ethical dilemmas), helping them translate insights into actionable changes in their practice.
- Support mentees in applying transformative insights, such as adopting new practices for compassionate care or enhancing inclusive team communication.

Continuous Feedback and Reflection

- Regularly provide timely, constructive feedback on clinical performance, research accomplishments, teaching ability, leadership development, and interpersonal skills.
- Invite mentees to regularly provide feedback on the mentorship process and adjust strategies accordingly.
- Conduct periodic mentoring check-ins dedicated to reviewing personal growth, clinical competencies, and career progress, adjusting goals as needed.

Mentorship-Led Innovation

In the best mentoring relationships, it is often hard to distinguish who is the mentor and who is the mentee. The curiosity and communication are fluid, ideas often bounce off one another, and both parties are actively growing. When such a mentoring relationship exists, there is clear psychological safety, which encourages experimentation, risk taking, and problem solving.[9] The person taking the risks doesn't fear retribution for any mistakes or omissions. When this environment is present, innovation occurs. This is how mentoring can lead to leadership. The innovation sparks a new line of thinking, project planning, and grant support, and someone needs to lead it all. See Worksheet 13.1 Leadership Innovation Reflection Guide for mentors and mentees to work together to identify opportunities for innovation.

Purpose

This professional guide supports mentors and mentees in collaboratively identifying and fostering opportunities for innovation within their healthcare mentorship relationship. It is designed to encourage **creative thinking**, **strategic experimentation**, and **continuous leadership development**.

Instructions

Complete each section together through **open** and **honest dialogue**. Clearly document your ideas and reflections to create actionable insights.

Step 1. Reflect on Current Practices

Clearly identify one or two specific processes or practices within your healthcare context (clinical, administrative, or educational) that could be enhanced through innovation:

1.

2.

Step 2. Opportunities for Innovation

Brainstorm and list concrete opportunities for innovation or experimentation connected to the practices identified above:

-
-
-

Step 3. Anticipating Barriers & Identifying Supports

Thoughtfully identify potential challenges you might face in implementing these innovations. Discuss how your mentorship relationship can actively address and overcome these barriers:

Barriers	Supports
•	•
•	•
•	•

WORKSHEET 13.1 Leadership Innovation Reflection Guide

Step 4. Leadership Roles & Responsibilities

Define clear roles and responsibilities for both mentor and mentee in pursuing the identified innovative opportunities:

Innovation Opportunity	Mentor Role	Mentee Role
1.		
2.		

Step 5. Action Plan & Timeline

Develop a detailed action plan, assigning clear responsibilities and establishing achievable timelines for implementing at least one innovation:

Action Step	Responsible Person	Due By
1.		
2.		

Step 6. Reflection & Follow-up

Schedule a structured follow-up meeting to review progress, discuss outcomes, and reflect on insights gained from the innovation process:

Scheduled Follow-up Date:

Reflections & Key Lessons Learned:

-
-
-

WORKSHEET 13.1 (Continued)

From Mentorship to Legacy Leadership

When all is said and done, people will remember less what you accomplished and more about those whose careers you shaped.[16] In other words, your legacy will be built and maintained by those you mentored. They will remember you, talk about you, and remind people about what you taught them and how you influenced their lives.

Techniques you devised, mnemonics you created, patient care principles you instilled, and professional values you inculcated in your mentees will live on, long after you leave the organization. They will be taught to the next generation, and have a ripple effect, all because you took on mentees and impacted their lives.

Summary

Mentorship and leadership are often intertwined but require distinct skills and roles, though it's not surprising that those who make good leaders often make good mentors. As job stability in healthcare declines, with physicians' and academic tenure becoming less common, the importance of mentors is growing. While leadership may often change, mentors remain a constant, guiding mentees through change and transition.

Mentor–leaders display four core competencies: trust, vision, empathy, and humility. Trust fosters commitment and collaboration, while vision encourages mentees to recognize their full potential. Empathy, grounded in shared experiences, creates deep understanding, and humility focuses on mentees' growth, instead of their own. Positive, energizing mentors do this through exhibiting virtuous behaviors like gratitude, kindness, and compassion. Effective mentorship is rooted in adult learning principles, emphasizing self-directed, experiential, and transformative learning. These principles support mentees in goal setting and skill development and foster innovation. Ultimately, mentors have an incredible opportunity to help shape their mentees and, through them, future generations. The legacy of a mentor lives on through the careers they shape.

Take-Home Points

- Effective mentors naturally exhibit leadership qualities such as trust, vision, empathy, and humility. While leadership positions may change frequently, mentors provide long-term guidance, becoming increasingly important as healthcare constantly evolves.
- Mentors provide continuity amidst change—whether it be in leadership, or the mentee's career path. Mentors help navigate transitions, support mentees in setting goals and developing skills, and encourage them to meet their full potential.
- Mentors build a legacy that impacts future generations. Through their influence, mentors contribute to shaping the achievements and careers of their mentees and of those that the mentees will one day guide.

14

Evaluating Mentoring Programs

Peter Drucker famously said, "What gets measured, gets managed."[1] If you are putting all the work into mentoring, how will you know if it is actually working? Having data points to prove the effectiveness of mentoring will help when you need to negotiate for resources, ranging from conference attendee fees to swag. Doing it systematically ensures you are delivering on negotiated objectives.

While we'll review some evaluation techniques and metrics, it is important to note that with mentoring, sometimes we won't see results for years, such as when you are working with someone to prepare them for a leadership role. It takes time to let the ideas and development marinate. Other times, the results may be intangible and therefore difficult to measure, such as improved confidence, decreased imposter syndrome, ideas on how to change an approach, key introductions, or reduced burnout. You need to differentiate between what is measurable and what is observable.

Determine What to Evaluate

As a first step, discuss the goals of mentoring with your mentee, and review what the metrics are to determine if the goals have been met. What can you observe as a measure that the goal has been achieved? Is it a conference presentation, a first-authored paper, improving technical skills (e.g., a new methodology or clinical procedure), or gaining confidence to speak up in lab meetings? Thinking about the skills and behaviors when developing goals and identifying success metrics will help both mentor and mentee recognize when the goal has been achieved.

DOI: 10.1201/9781003611233-17

Differentiating between overt and covert skills and behaviors will help you zero in on what to evaluate. Some common areas for evaluation for both individual and group mentoring programs and related examples include:

- **Satisfaction and engagement:** High satisfaction ratings from mentees on mentoring experience surveys.

- **Self-confidence and self-efficacy:** Improved confidence in trying things previously avoided or approached with trepidation. Greater willingness to try things outside of their comfort zone.

- **Career profession and professional development:** Increased percentage of mentees achieving promotions, leadership roles within the organization or national society, presentations, published manuscripts, or grants. Increase in their professional network.

- **Clinical competency and skill advancement:** Measurable improvement in procedural or diagnostic skills and clinical decision making.

- **Retention rates:** Decreased turnover rates among nursing staff and junior attendings who participated in the mentoring program.

- **Burnout prevention and improved clinician well-being:** Reduction in burnout symptoms and absenteeism and improved work–life balance scores among those who participated in the mentoring program.

- **Enhanced patient outcomes:** Measurable improvements in patient safety, reduction in medication errors, and higher patient satisfaction scores linked directly to clinicians involved in mentoring.

Observable Indicators of Success

Certain changes in behavior are more observable and might be difficult to quantify. While they might be subtle, if you start to add them all up, they show an improvement in the mentee. You might observe their increased attendance at non-mandatory meetings or gatherings and coming more prepared for mentoring sessions. You start to notice their increased confidence and proactive leadership. Perhaps they start to ask questions and speak up in research meetings or Grand Rounds, when previously, they rarely asked a question. They might also start to take charge of things ranging from coffee runs to managing the group's Slack channel. Perhaps they take on greater leadership initiative and organize a grant review process or schedule practice talks with everyone before a conference. They become active participants instead of passive observers in their career development journey.

As you notice these changes, others might as well. Colleagues and supervisors might comment on the positive change in the mentee's personal and professional communication and interactions. The mentee themselves might recognize their improved self-confidence when they start handling complex clinical scenarios and, on reflection, recognize that they handled the challenges well.

Evaluation Methods

Beyond the observations, there are varying ways to measure the effectiveness of mentoring, and they range from qualitative to quantitative, and often to a mixture of both methods.

Quantitative Evaluations

Surveys are a great, quick way to get the pulse of what is happening. The answers are often yes/no or on a Likert scale. Some potential questions to ask the mentee include:

1. How satisfied are you with the mentoring you are receiving?
2. How comfortable do you feel sharing personal concerns (housing, financial, family, physical/mental health)?
3. How comfortable do you feel sharing professional concerns (papers, grants, talks, lab meetings, call schedule, fund of knowledge, board exams, etc.)?
4. Do you feel you are working more hours than necessary?
5. Do you feel pressure to avoid taking days off/vacation?
6. Do you feel empowered to make suggestions or take on a new challenge?
7. Do you feel you are getting enough feedback?
8. Do you feel you are meeting with me enough?
9. How effective do you feel the meetings are?
10. Do you feel you are learning career skills in addition to clinical/basic science skills?
11. Did you publish any papers this year? How many?
12. Did you present any talks this year? How many?
13. Did you get any grants this year? How many?
14. Did you receive any awards this year? How many?

Quantitative surveys of this kind are adequate for tracking career progression and promotional achievements. It's also easier to analyze this data. The challenge with these yes/no questions is that they are what are often referred to as closed questions. They don't provide an opportunity to dig beyond the answers. It's almost impossible to get to the "why" behind certain answers with such closed responses. For example, if a mentee feels overworked and doesn't feel they can take a day off, it would be helpful to understand what is driving that line of thinking and feeling. Is the mentor subconsciously sending a signal that working long hours is expected, and taking days off is seen as a sign of being uncommitted? These questions cannot be answered on a standard quantitative survey alone.

Qualitative Evaluations

Qualitative evaluations help answer the "why" behind responses. They are open-ended questions, which allow the mentee to go deeper with their responses. Traditional qualitative evaluations include interviews, observations, narrative reflections, and journaling. Perhaps the easiest approach is to add an open-ended question at the end of a survey in which you ask the respondent to provide feedback on the mentoring team or mentoring meeting and ask whether they have anything else to add. When interviews are held in person, follow-up questions to go deeper into a subject is a popular strategy.

Mentor–Mentee Feedback

When doing in-person interviews, behavioral questions, which require the mentee to give a particular example, are often a useful opportunity for greater inquiry. Some good questions to ask are:

1. How did your mentor help you achieve your clinical/research goals?
2. What was the most impactful guidance your mentor provided?
3. In what ways has your mentor influenced your clinical/research decision-making process?
4. Take me through the development of your research project. How did you develop your hypothesis? How did you discuss this with your mentor? How did they help you formulate the hypothesis, frame your research questions, understand the outcomes of your study, and present your findings in both an oral and written format?

Dr. Stephen Brookfield recommends using a Critical Incident Questionnaire,[2] which focuses on four main questions (adapted by the book authors for purposes of mentoring):

1. At what moment during your mentoring discussions were you most engaged by what was happening? Why?
2. At what moment during your mentoring discussions were you most distanced from the conversation? Why?
3. What action did your mentor take that you found most affirming or helpful?
4. What action did your mentor take that you found most puzzling or confusing?
5. What was something your mentor said or did that took you by surprise?

Individual Interview Questions

Without it sounding like an interrogation, you can let your mentee know that you are always looking to improve and refine your mentoring skills. Then rework the mentor–mentee feedback questions into first person.

At Rockefeller University, principal investigator Dr. Vanessa Ruda developed an anonymous lab survey,[3] which was then expanded upon and shared publicly[4] by another Rockefeller scientist, Dr. Leslie Vosshall, who is also the vice president and chief scientific officer of the Howard Hughes Medical Institute. By annually requesting feedback from the trainees, the heads of labs, who are mentors to their students and postdocs, are getting real-time insights into what is working and what is not.

With both the Critical Incident Questionnaire and the Anonymous Lab Survey, it is important to look for themes and differentiate those from noise. If several people are saying it's hard to get focused time with you, start listening. If one person is saying it, you don't need to run and cancel cases and rework your entire calendar.

Group Interview Questions

Focus groups, which in essence are structured group interviews, can be a useful tool in evaluations. While a mentee might not come to a realization on their own, they might when someone else brings up a scenario or feeling. This way, conversations build off one another, and an otherwise quiet mentee might be more willing to share. This is an especially helpful exercise if someone other than the mentor takes the lead in asking questions.

This format allows people to build off one another's answers in a psychologically safe manner. Results are then de-identified and shared as themes, thereby keeping individual responses anonymous.

Some questions to ask during this group evaluation are:

1. What was something helpful that occurred as a result of your mentoring?
2. Was there anything in mentoring that derailed your progress?
3. In what way did participating in mentoring influence your collaboration with colleagues?

This format, along with its benefits, however, runs the risk of "group think"—the idea that thinking or decision making is done as a group in a way that discourages individual thinking, responsibility, and creativity.[5] A way of overcoming this is to have a skilled facilitator to ensure that no one person dominates the conversation or imposes undue influence on the group with the goal of getting their way. The goal of the group interview is to uncover some truths, not create a revolt.

Journaling

Journaling is a popular mode of reflection. It allows the mentee to write what they did and what is on their mind and in their heart. Reflective journaling has been shown to help develop critical thinking.[6] This type of reflective exercise can be done by the mentor or mentee privately or, with permission, shared with others.

Three issues with journaling need to be considered. First, not everyone can reflect on command, especially extroverts.[7] They may need more time for ideas to marinate. Second, reflection only works if you go back to it, look for emerging themes, and then take action. The learning happens when that last step, action, is taken. Finally, while journaling may help the mentee reflect, if the ideas aren't shared, the mentor is left in the dark as to what is and is not working.

Yet journaling is extremely popular, and many find it very useful. To increase its usefulness, you may wish to guide the mentee with some prompts:

1. Reflect on a time when your mentor's advice significantly impacted your X, Y, Z. What was said? What happened?
2. Describe a way in which you feel you grew in your clinical/research skills. Did your confidence improve? Are you able to do things now that you couldn't do six months ago?

Mixed-Methods Approach

Perhaps the most rigorous approach is a mixed-methods approach: part quantitative survey and part open-ended questions to elicit qualitative information. Like any research, evaluations are best when the data is "triangulated." Looking at surveys, interviews, and other data—including how many papers or presentations were given or grants awarded to the people under your tutelage—will offer a picture as to the effectiveness of your mentorship and the opportunities for enhancement.

Presenting the "Return on Investment" of Mentorship

If you have results that showcase your effective mentorship, don't keep them a secret. Showcase them and make them part of your brand. Include them on your lab webpage and share them with your chair or dean. If you become the "pied piper" of mentoring—the mentor who has influenced many careers—show the numbers. Consider creating an infographic that showcases the benefits of your mentoring. It becomes part of your ethos.

Nearly every laboratory has a "lab handbook,"[8] which can be found on their website. It codifies the lab's techniques, culture, expectations, and roles. It ensures everyone is on the same page regarding work hours, productivity expectations, and communication styles. This helps someone new, who is entering the group, understand the ethos of the laboratory. It's especially helpful as it removes the stress of the "hidden curriculum"—the nuanced behaviors and expectations that everyone is supposed to know but no one tells them.[9]

The lab notebook can also showcase the benefits of being a member of your lab. It shares the accomplishments of lab members. It tells a story that, if you want to succeed, this is the lab to be in, not because of endless resources but rather because the mentorship is life-altering.

Proven Programs

This section outlines two structured mentoring programs—one for busy clinicians and one for research-oriented faculty—detailing their components, outcomes, and evaluation methods.

Mentoring Program for Clinicians

Clinician educators are less likely to receive mentorship than physician-scientists, according to a prior prevalence study.[10] Recognizing the unique challenges faced by clinicians striving for academic advancement, a team at a midwestern Veterans' Affairs tertiary care medical center, led by Dr. Nathan Houchens, established a committee mentoring program and studied its efficacy.[11] This systematic mentoring approach was designed with the goal not only to facilitate career progression but also to enhance job satisfaction and reduce burnout.

The program focused on faculty members within the Medicine Service who were below the rank of clinical associate professor. For each mentee involved in the study, a mentoring committee was established, which consisted of three to six committee mentors and one chair chosen by the mentee. Mentees personally identified and requested mentor involvement via email, with assistance as needed from a dedicated project manager.

Twice-annual mentoring meetings brought together the mentee, chair, and all committee members. Meetings were led by the mentee and committee chair, and covered the short-, middle-, and long-term goals of the mentee. Their progression since the last meeting was reviewed, along with job satisfaction and mentors' suggestions for advancement. Time was also allotted for the mentee to provide feedback to the committee on how he or she could be more effectively mentored or sponsored. This design ensured a consistent and comprehensive support structure, with robust engagement from all participants contributing to the program's success.

As each meeting concluded, a standardized survey instrument called the Mentoring Meeting Assessment Tool (MMAT) was distributed to all participants[11] (see Worksheet 14.1 for a copy of this tool). The electronic survey used Likert-scale questions to obtain information regarding the logistics of the meeting and whether it was considered an effective use of time. Additionally, participants were asked to score perceptions of effectiveness, clarity on next steps, sense of progress since the last meeting, and impacts of the program on satisfaction and burnout. Response to the MMAT from all participants was 100%. Of the 23 enrolled clinical faculty members, 3 (13%) were promoted to clinical associate professor, and the remaining 20 (87%) chose to continue in the program.

Thus the study yielded highly encouraging results. Participants consistently rated the program positively across multiple facets, including effective use of time, appropriate progress from one meeting to the next, and improvements in work satisfaction and burnout alleviation. Among the *mentors*, 98% indicated the meetings were an effective use of time, 99% agreed feedback provided was received positively by the mentee, and 94% agreed the mentee made appropriate progress since the prior meeting and that the next steps were clear. The majority of mentors also agreed that the program increased their job satisfaction and reduced their level of burnout.

Among *mentees*, 90% or more agreed that committee meetings were an effective use of time, that they were comfortable raising issues with mentors, and that the next steps were clear. Likewise, the majority of mentees also agreed that the program increased their job satisfaction and reduced their level of burnout.

These outcomes demonstrate that structured mentorship targeting physicians on the clinical track not only supports the tangible aspects of career development—such as promotions—but also significantly enhances the intangible elements like confidence, work satisfaction, and overall well-being. By carefully aligning mentoring efforts with clearly defined objectives and metrics, the program offers a potential blueprint for fostering success in clinical academia, highlighting the impact of structured mentorship.

Given the success of this program for junior faculty, the program has now been expanded to include those in mid-career who have not reached the rank of full professor. Such a program is consistent with what others have done, labeling such programs as "Boost" teams or committees.[12]

Mentoring Program for Clinical Researchers

High-quality research that positively impacts patient lives is essential to advancing patient care. The US Department of Veterans Affairs Office of Research and Development places a strong emphasis on this priority, as demonstrated by nearly a century of groundbreaking studies conducted by VA researchers.

Navigating grant writing, funding, and research design requires experienced mentorship, yet clinical researchers often face barriers like time constraints, competing priorities, and lack of resources. In response, the VA Ann Arbor Healthcare System launched a Clinical Research Mentorship Program in 2015.[13] This program helps junior clinical investigators develop and submit research grant applications through group mentorship

1. Please enter your name _____

2. Please enter your role (select only one option)
   - ☐ Mentee
   - ☐ Mentoring committee chair
   - ☐ Mentoring committee member

3. Please enter the mentee's name _____ **(MENTORS ONLY)**

4. Please enter the date of the meeting _____ **(MENTEES ONLY)**

5. Mentee's CV was sent to all mentors before the meeting **(MENTORS ONLY)**
   - ☐ Yes
   - ☐ No

6. The meeting began on time
   - ☐ Yes
   - ☐ No

7. Sufficient time was allotted for the meeting
   - ☐ Strongly agree
   - ☐ Agree
   - ☐ Neither agree nor disagree
   - ☐ Disagree
   - ☐ Strongly disagree

8. Overall, the meeting was an effective use of my time
   - ☐ Strongly agree
   - ☐ Agree
   - ☐ Neither agree nor disagree
   - ☐ Disagree
   - ☐ Strongly disagree

9. I discussed _____ action items I wanted to during the meeting **(MENTEES ONLY)**
   - ☐ All
   - ☐ Most
   - ☐ Some
   - ☐ Few
   - ☐ No

10. I felt comfortable raising issues with mentors **(MENTEES ONLY)**
    - ☐ Strongly agree
    - ☐ Agree
    - ☐ Neither agree nor disagree
    - ☐ Disagree
    - ☐ Strongly disagree

11. Feedback given by mentors was specific, actionable, and focused on how to improve **(MENTEES ONLY)**
    - ☐ Strongly agree
    - ☐ Agree
    - ☐ Neither agree nor disagree
    - ☐ Disagree
    - ☐ Strongly disagree

12. Feedback given by mentors was received in a positive manner by mentee **(MENTORS ONLY)**
    - ☐ Strongly agree
    - ☐ Agree
    - ☐ Neither agree nor disagree
    - ☐ Disagree
    - ☐ Strongly disagree

WORKSHEET 14.1 Mentoring Meeting Assessment Tool

Source: This worksheet is reprinted from "Committed to Success: A Structured Mentoring Program for Clinically Oriented Physicians" (Houchens N, Kuhn L, Ratz D, Su GL, & Saint S), published in Mayo Clinic Proceedings: Innovations, Quality & Outcomes (2024, https://doi.org/10.1016/j.mayocpiqo.2024.05.002), under a Creative Commons Attribution 4.0 International License (CC BY 4.0, https://creativecommons.org/licenses/by/4.0/). No content changes were made.

13. I trust that my mentors are committed to my professional success   **(MENTEES ONLY)**
    - ☐ Strongly agree
    - ☐ Agree
    - ☐ Neither agree nor disagree
    - ☐ Disagree
    - ☐ Strongly disagree

14. My mentors are helping me set and achieve career goals   **(MENTEES ONLY)**
    - ☐ Strongly agree
    - ☐ Agree
    - ☐ Neither agree nor disagree
    - ☐ Disagree
    - ☐ Strongly disagree .

15. At the end of the meeting, next steps were clear (i.e., who is doing what by when)
    - ☐ Strongly agree
    - ☐ Agree
    - ☐ Neither agree nor disagree
    - ☐ Disagree
    - ☐ Strongly disagree

16. Overall, this mentoring program has increased my level of satisfaction with my work
    - ☐ Strongly agree
    - ☐ Agree
    - ☐ Neither agree nor disagree
    - ☐ Disagree
    - ☐ Strongly disagree

17. Overall, this mentoring program has reduced my level of burnout (e.g., exhaustion, depersonalization, and/or reduced achievement) from my work
    - ☐ Strongly agree
    - ☐ Agree
    - ☐ Neither agree nor disagree
    - ☐ Disagree
    - ☐ Strongly disagree

Please provide additional comments:

WORKSHEET 14.1 (Continued)

and one-on-one services provided by two experienced program directors. Additional support is available as needed from a statistician, program coordinator, epidemiologist, and research assistant. The program encourages peer mentorship through participant feedback during group meetings, which are held bimonthly during the nine-month academic period.

Recruitment involves annual emails to faculty and leaders inviting applications. Applicants submit a Curriculum Vitae (CV) and a one-page summary of research area interests, relevancy to the VA, and a proposed research study concept, design, and significance. Applications are reviewed by the two program directors and program coordinator based on research focus, training, past success, funding potential, and research availability. Typically, 90% of applicants are invited to participate in the program.

Meetings, held in person and via Zoom, do not enforce attendance, allowing mentees to join as their schedule permits. Ahead of the meetings, the program coordinator solicits agenda items from members. Mentees then present their research ideas and updates, and program directors facilitate open group discussions providing strategic feedback and tackling emerging challenges. Grant-specific concerns, research procedures, manuscript or presentation preparation, and career-related issues were common discussion points. This setting encouraged mentees to refine research projects, receive constructive criticism, learn from faculty mentors, and develop peer mentorship practices such as collective problem solving and peer support.

Since the initiation of the program in 2015, 35 clinician researchers have participated. Thirty-three grant proposals have been submitted, and as of 2024, 19 (58%) have been funded. Aside from funding success, participants annually complete an end-of-year survey evaluating the mentorship program. Survey responses show that the majority of program participants agreed that these meetings were an effective use of their time, that they were able to discuss most items they wanted to address during the meetings, that the program helped them set and achieve their research goals, and that feedback received during meetings was actionable and helped improve their research agenda. An increase in work satisfaction, along with reduced levels of burnout, were also reported by more than half of the participants.

These findings illustrate the substantial benefits of facilitated group discussion and peer mentorship for clinician researchers. By fostering a collaborative learning environment and providing consistent support and guidance, the program has helped participants develop valuable research skills and accelerate their professional growth, while empowering mentees to better support and mentor one another. This program can serve as a model for other VA or non-VA academic medical centers which focus on developing research faculty.

Summary

Evaluating your mentorship provides insight into what is going well and what isn't, and when you need to adapt. Systematically tracking mentoring outcomes and fulfilling objectives also allow for better resource negotiation, and proves your time is being used effectively. But proper evaluations must differentiate between intangible results, such as improved confidence or reduced burnout, and what can be quantitatively measured, like publications or promotions. The first step involves defining mentoring goals with mentees and establishing clear metrics for their achievement. A comprehensive evaluation should employ a mixed-methods approach—combining quantitative surveys, qualitative feedback, and observable success indicators. Structured group mentorship programs in clinical and research settings may provide a thorough mentorship approach, targeting tangible aspects of career development and enhancing job satisfaction, confidence, and peer support. By aligning goals and methodologies, these programs may serve as blueprints for fostering professional growth and well-being in healthcare.

Take-Home Points

- Mentorship yields both immediate and long-term benefits, some of which are difficult to quantify. Improved self-confidence, well-being, and job satisfaction may not be easily measured, though growth in these areas often becomes clear over time. Effective mentorship promotes more than just the observable metrics of success.
- A triangulated evaluation—including quantitative surveys, open-ended qualitative questions, and quantifiable metrics of success (such as publications, or grants awarded)—offers the fullest picture of your mentorship. Look for ways to incorporate all three.
- Following the approach of structured mentoring programs may accelerate professional growth and provide measurable outcomes for a group of mentees. Approaches tailored to the mentees' track (clinical or research-oriented) are available and have been shown to be effective.

15

Mindfulness in the Mentorship Relationship

It was a normal chaotic day in a U.S. Senate office. I had recently started a new job as a press aide on Capitol Hill. I was only 23 and felt inexperienced, intimidated around senior staffers and members of Congress. I wasn't sure I could handle the job. To add to my anxiety, that morning we were told the Senator wanted to issue an immediate press release on a news story. My supervisor, who later became a lifelong mentor to me, was unfazed as a seasoned press secretary. He looked at me and said, "You write this one and handle the reporters today." He must have seen the terror in my eyes as up until then, I had only watched him do these things. He walked over to me, sat down, smiled reassuringly, and said, "Listen, you're a good, fast writer, and I know you can handle this. I trust you. Sometimes you just have to jump in." He held my gaze for awhile, and I finally said "okay." I did indeed jump in—and learned that I could handle it. That moment and my mentor's faith in me gave me the courage and self-confidence I was lacking and was a turning point for me. To this day, when unsure, I remind myself to just "jump in."

—**Martha Quinn, MPH, University of
Michigan School of Public Health**

That brief yet powerful moment of encouragement transformed this mentee's self-doubt into confidence. It became a turning point in her career, illustrating the profound impact a mentor's trust, support, and encouragement can have on a mentee. As we will discuss later in this chapter, it was perhaps even a "sacred moment"[1] in the mentoring relationship, given its long-lasting effect on at least one of the participants. Such a deep moment

DOI: 10.1201/9781003611233-18

of connection helps us get to the essence of "mindful mentorship," where empathy and belief in a mentee's potential catalyze growth and self-discovery. As we will discuss further in this chapter, mentors guide not merely with their technical expertise and know-how but, as importantly, with a heartful human connection that hopefully resonates both personally and professionally with the mentee. In this chapter, we explore how mindfulness serves as a foundational element in enhancing mentoring relationships, encouraging both parties to be fully present, empathetic, and attuned to each other's needs, goals, and aspirations.

Understanding Mindfulness in Mentoring

Mindfulness, with origins dating back over 2,500 years to the Eastern religions of Hinduism and Buddhism, is about maintaining an openness, patience, and acceptance while remaining non-judgmentally focused on the unfolding situation. Readers may be familiar with the concept of mindfulness during meditation or while walking, but mindfulness has been used and studied in a variety of contexts including while washing hands in the hospital.[2] In a mentoring context, mindfulness extends beyond scientific expertise and methodological skills, fostering a connection where mentors guide the mentee with care, compassion, and understanding.[3] It offers a holistic approach that prioritizes the well-being and development of mentees, allowing for the cultivation of selfless and authentic relationships. Indeed, many argue that mindfulness and heartfulness are closely intertwined and that truly mindful mentors lead with both head and heart.[4]

Mentors who can remain mindful and non-judgmental during mentoring sessions, unsurprisingly, are the types of mentors whom mentees trust, tend to listen to, and look forward to meeting with. Such mentoring shifts the emphasis from exclusively focusing on rigid academic metrics such as papers written, grants submitted, or clinical work completed (all of which remain important to success, of course) to nurturing professional growth, sparking creativity, and considering higher-risk, more impactful projects. Such a shift can lead to unexpected and groundbreaking results. Mindfulness also alters the perspective of mentoring from a chore to a source of energy and joy,[5] positively impacting organizational culture by embedding values of empathy and authenticity. Finally, using mindfulness helps prevent mentors from committing mentorship malpractice;[6] similarly, it aids mentees in avoiding missteps.[7]

Putting Yourself in the Shoes of Your Mentee

Mindful mentorship requires a deep understanding and empathy toward a mentee's perspective. To truly assist and uplift, mentors must step into the mentee's shoes, embracing the challenges, fears, and aspirations they hold. This empathic approach fosters a nurturing environment and builds trust—integral for effective mentorship.

In the Senate office anecdote, the mentor didn't simply assign a task and walk away. Instead, the mentor recognized the mentee's inexperience and fear, yet chose to empower her by expressing trust and seeing the potential she couldn't yet see in herself. This act of understanding and reassurance exemplifies what it means to empathize with a mentee's situation.

To effectively put oneself in a mentee's shoes, mentors must recall their own early career fears and challenges. Sharing experiences of struggle can demystify the path of growth, reframing failures as valuable learning experiences. This humanizes mentors, making them more relatable and approachable. Mentors tend to be quite successful professionally; thus some may forget what it is like to feel vulnerable as a junior person. Truly imagining what it is like to be dependent, for example, on obtaining a career development grant to launch an academic career or publishing a high-impact paper required for promotion can help the mentor see things from the mentee's perspective and better understand the anxiety the mentee may be experiencing.

Creating a safe space for mentees to express such concerns, uncertainties, and anxieties is paramount. Mentors who practice empathy and active listening[8] foster a relationship where mentees feel valued and understood. By embracing the mentee's viewpoint and encouraging open dialogue, mentors empower them not only to develop professionally but also personally, standing by them as they navigate their journeys.

The mindfulness practices embedded in this approach to mentorship benefit both the mentor and the mentee. Building relationships on foundations of empathy and genuine care allows mentors and mentees to connect and craft legacies of mutual support and profound impact beyond conventional achievements. Through mindful mentorship, mentors become catalysts for unlocking potential and resilience, guiding mentees to envision and achieve possibilities they might not have imagined on their own, as in the example that began this chapter. Importantly, such an approach also models to the mentee what a successful mindfulness-based mentoring relationship may look like. In this way, the mentee may employ a similar approach when it is their opportunity to serve as a mentor—which happens surprisingly quickly in healthcare settings, whether in the clinical setting[9] or in a research role.

Motivational Interviewing as a Way to Connect

"Motivational interviewing" is a patient-centered approach for enhancing intrinsic motivation to change by exploring and resolving ambivalence. Originally developed in the context of addiction counseling, motivational interviewing has been applied to various fields, including education, organizational leadership, and healthcare.[10] While this technique is typically used by clinicians for patients to guide behavior change when a patient is uncertain about what to do, ambivalent behavioral patterns are not limited to patients. Motivational interviewing can play a pivotal role in a mentoring relationship by encouraging mentees to articulate their goals, identify barriers, and develop actionable strategies for change.

At its core, motivational interviewing is based on four key principles: (1) expressing empathy, (2) discerning discrepancy, (3) recognizing resistance, and (4) supporting self-efficacy.[11] In a mentoring context, these principles help create a supportive environment where mentees feel understood and motivated to pursue their aspirations. By expressing empathy, mentors can build a trusting relationship, making mentees feel heard and valued. This empathetic approach is essential for establishing a safe space for open dialogue, which is crucial for effective mentoring. Mindfulness, of course, helps ensure such psychological safety in the relationship.[12]

Discerning discrepancy involves helping mentees recognize the gap between their current behavior (e.g., not completing a manuscript or grant by a certain deadline) and their broader goals or values (e.g., obtaining a competitive academic job offer). In a mentoring relationship, this principle can be applied to guide mentees in reflecting on their career paths, personal development, or specific challenges they face. By gently highlighting these discrepancies, mentors can inspire mentees to consider changes that align with their long-term objectives, thereby promoting self-awareness and intentional growth.

Recognizing resistance is another critical aspect of motivational interviewing that can enhance mentoring. Rather than confronting or opposing a mentee's resistance to change, mentors using motivational interviewing techniques acknowledge and explore it. This approach prevents defensiveness and encourages mentees to express their concerns and hesitations openly. By understanding the roots of resistance, mentors can collaboratively explore alternative perspectives and solutions, ultimately empowering mentees to overcome their obstacles. Importantly, the mentor should view themselves as partnering with the mentee to achieve the mentee's goals rather than simply telling the mentee what to do.

Supporting self-efficacy,[13] or the belief in one's ability to succeed, is foundational in both motivational interviewing and mentoring. Encouraging this belief involves recognizing and reinforcing a mentee's strengths and achievements, which can boost their confidence and motivation to tackle challenges as in the anecdote that opened this chapter. In a mentoring relationship, mentors can utilize motivational interviewing techniques to help mentees identify past successes and apply these experiences to current goals. This empowerment fosters a sense of agency and resilience, critical for personal and professional development.

The collaborative nature of motivational interviewing aligns well with the dynamics of a mentoring relationship, where both mentor and mentee actively engage in the process of exploration and growth. Most importantly, motivational interviewing encourages mentors to adopt a non-directive approach, allowing mentees to drive the conversation and solution-finding process. This empowers mentees to take ownership of their development, fostering independence and intrinsic motivation. Incorporating motivational interviewing into mentoring also enhances communication skills, for both mentors and mentees. The reflective listening and open-ended questioning techniques that are intrinsic to motivational interviewing encourage deeper understanding and clarity. These skills not only improve the quality of the mentoring relationship but also equip mentees with valuable interpersonal skills applicable in various aspects of their lives. We've created Worksheet 15.1 to get you started on applying motivational interviewing in mentoring.

The Power of Sacred Moments

When mindful mentors use the techniques of motivational interviewing, the environment created may allow for sacred moments to occur. Sacred

Purpose

This professional guide supports mentors when applying motivational interviewing techniques to help their mentees clarify their goals and develop (or uncover) their own motivation.

Instructions

Mentors can use this worksheet to apply motivational interviewing techniques during mentoring conversations.

Step 1. Express Empathy

✓ Acknowledge emotion

"That sounds frustrating. I can understand why you feel that way."

"It sounds like this is something you care about deeply."

"Having experienced that myself, I get how hard that is to deal with."

✗ Avoid dismissing concerns

Try, "Tell me more about what's challenging you," *instead of,* "Just push through it."

Try, "Let's walk through the issues you're facing," *instead of,* "You're going to have to figure this out."

"You've mentioned worries about [X] several times. Do you want to work through that together?"

What emotions is my mentee expressing?

_____

_____

How can I validate their experience?

_____

_____

Step 2. Discern Discrepancy

✓ Highlight gaps between goals (and/or values) and current actions

"You mentioned wanting [goal]. How do you see your current situation aligning with that goal?"

What are my mentee's long-term goals?

_____

_____

Where does my mentee see misalignment?

_____

_____

WORKSHEET 15.1 Applying Motivational Interviewing in Mentoring

Step 3. Recognize Resistance

✗ Avoid arguing when mentee demonstrates resistance—*Ask guiding questions, instead:*

"What do you think is getting in the way?"
"What has worked for you in the past?"

What resistance is my mentee expressing?

_____

_____

How can I help my mentee explore alternatives?

_____

_____

Step 4. Support Self-Efficacy

✓ Identify (if needed) & reinforce strengths
"You've done this before. What helped you succeed then?"

✓ Encourage small steps
"What's one thing you can do this week to move forward?"

What strengths does my mentee demonstrate?

_____

_____

What is one actionable step my mentee can take to make progress?

_____

_____

WORKSHEET 15.1 (Continued)

moments—a term used more in the psychological than in the spiritual sense—was coined by Ken Pargament when describing deep and meaningful connections between clinical psychologists and patients.[1] Sacred moments can be considered brief periods when time seems to stand still, and a deep understanding is achieved. Sacred moments have been described among musicians,[14] in the acute care hospital setting,[15] among radiation oncology clinicians,[16] and in the context of mentoring.[17] Indeed, these moments of profound connection offer clarity, reassurance, and encouragement, allowing mentees to recognize their potential beyond perceived failures.

Sacred moments build trust and lasting bonds not only by addressing the immediate challenges but by reshaping self-perception and inspiring confidence. Dr. Suzanne Koven's assertion that a mentor is "someone with more imagination about you than you have about yourself"[18] encapsulates the transformative power of these interactions and how mentors can help alter a mentee's trajectory. These moments have been described as instrumental in defining careers, where mentors provided not just guidance but affirmation that encouraged significant personal and professional strides.[17]

Practices for Mindful Mentorship

To cultivate mindfulness during a mentoring relationship, mentors can use the following five practices to enhance interactions with mentees:

1. **Self-reflection:** Mentors should begin by asking themselves why they spend their time mentoring. By connecting with their motivations and reflecting on what they gain from the experience, mentors can align their intentions with actions. This self-awareness fosters a genuine commitment to the mentee's journey and encourages openness to both successes and failures.

2. **Empathy and perspective taking:** As previously touched on, it's crucial for mentors to place themselves in their mentee's shoes, recognizing the mentee's challenges and aspirations. By choosing words carefully and sharing personal experiences, mentors can reduce the pressure of judgment, building a nurturing environment where mistakes are seen as opportunities for learning.

3. **Present-moment engagement:** Mindful mentors prioritize being totally present. By setting aside distractions, they fully engage with their

mentee, creating a space for connection. This presence allows for curiosity and understanding, making it easier to address underlying issues that are central to growth. This will, of course, require putting the smartphone down and not multitasking when meeting with the mentee, whether it be in person, virtually, or over the phone.

4. **Gratitude:** Feeling and expressing gratitude reinforces a positive mentoring dynamic. Recognizing the mentee's contributions, acknowledging their efforts, and expressing appreciation for the shared journey foster mutual respect and encourage a cycle of gratitude that permeates the mentor–mentee relationship.

5. **Selflessness:** Embracing selflessness means focusing on the mentee's development, guiding them to unlock their full potential. This involves restraint in directing conversations and projects, allowing mentees to emerge as leaders in their own right. Using these motivational interviewing techniques will allow this to happen.

Challenges and Considerations

Mindful mentorship is not without its challenges. Adopting mindfulness practices may require mentors to step outside their comfort zones, especially if it involves confronting inadequate non-verbal communication or addressing cultural nuances in mentorship dynamics. Remaining non-judgmental during an unfolding situation is not easy. Similarly, refraining from being overly directive—as motivational interviewing would recommend—comes only with practice. Indeed, some mentors might feel the discomfort of inadequacy when not providing direct solutions to a mentee's problems, making it essential for mentors to find a balance between directing and gently nudging. As well, mentees may feel that a mentor is not providing clear directions, and resistance may come from mentees unaccustomed to this approach. Too often, mentees may wish simply to be told what to do and how to do it. While such an approach may help in the short run, it will stunt a mentee's development in the long run. Being clear about the fact that you would like the mentee to help develop solutions is, in fact, part of being mindful and heartful. Establishing a mutual understanding of what mindfulness looks like in the relationship certainly may take time and adaptation. However, the deep, meaningful connections forged through a mindful approach invariably outweigh these initial hurdles.

Summary

Integrating mindfulness into mentorship relationships offers a pathway to transformative growth, not only enhancing individual mentorship experiences but potentially reshaping the culture of academic and professional environments. Mindful mentors are typically adept at deploying the key tenets of motivational interviewing: (1) expressing empathy, (2) discerning discrepancies, (3) recognizing resistance, and (4) supporting mentee self-efficacy. In a mentoring context, relying on these principles coupled with practical mindfulness approaches—self-reflection, empathy, present-moment engagement, and being both grateful and selfless—helps create a supportive environment where mentees feel understood and motivated to pursue their aspirations. Through mindfulness, mentors and mentees alike can create sacred moments that transcend traditional metrics and lead to meaningful encounters.

Take-Home Points

- Mindful mentorship entails self-reflection, empathy, gratitude, engaging in the present moment, and selflessness, which cultivate meaningful mentor–mentee interactions. Despite the effort it may take to step out of your comfort zone, the personal connection created is rewarding for both you and your mentee.

- Motivational interviewing encourages mentees to articulate goals and overcome challenges; this approach may lead to transformative encounters that impact the mentee's career path and personal growth.

- As a mentor, you offer not only career advice but personal connection. Being mindful in your mentorship creates a supportive environment that fosters growth, confidence, and self-discovery for mentees.

16

Looking Back While Traveling Forward

Mentorship is a privilege; it's also not a life sentence. We thought it prudent to close with some parting words of wisdom by reflecting on how best to operationalize the guidance in these pages while simultaneously looking forward to what the future holds.

Looking Back

If you are new to mentoring someone, you may feel anxious or uneasy about the responsibility. That's a good sign, as it means you understand the importance mentorship plays in both your professional career and your field. Furthermore, mentoring someone—or being mentored by someone—who is different from you can feel challenging. Our hope is that the wisdom in this book makes this task less formidable and greatly enjoyable.

When it comes to finding an ideal mentor, perfection is unattainable.[1] Our advice is that mentors, especially those who are new to this role of guiding others, should not harbor unrealistic expectations of themselves or their mentees. Beware of placing unnecessary burdens on yourself to ensure that your first experience is successful.

The same holds true for a brand-new employee, a junior faculty member, or a new staff member in a new organization. Without knowing anyone, the search for a mentor amid the unknown can be paralyzing. The decision is not insignificant as mentees are fully aware that if chosen correctly, a new mentor can open professional doors and be crucial to their success.

As previously discussed, not having a mentor can really hinder your career. In the academic world as well as in many corporate organizations, lack of high-quality mentorship can set you back years and make the professional ascension longer and harder than necessary.

For many, including the authors of this book, receiving the guidance of a mentor and then serving to help others has been transformative. These experiences gave us much needed additional perspectives and enriched our lives and our views of the world. In fact, each of us shares immense gratitude to our individual mentors and mentoring teams for guiding us and accompanying us on the journey to our current positions. We can identify exact words they used at critical junctures that led to certain decisions we made. There were some bumps in the road, which at times seemed insurmountable, but the mentors always saw things we couldn't quite recognize yet. Trust and their belief in each of us allowed us to stay the course.

The flip side is equally exciting, if not more so. We have each experienced the deep satisfaction and pure joy that comes when our mentee has been recognized for their abilities and talents and rose to positions of influence. We have even benefited from this as our mentees have served as guides to us as we take on new challenges or opportunities. This is the circle of life and of mentorship at work. After all, the world has changed over time, so we find ourselves learning from our mentees as much as they learn from us—as it should be. We gain insight into the challenges our mentees encounter, many of which differ from those we experienced. Whether related to professional conflicts, balancing work with life, or dealing with toxic mentors, we listen with great interest and care.

Every successful CEO and industry leader shares the same respect and admiration for the mentoring relationships that helped them get to where they are now. In fact, they often share that what they missed the most as they ascended to leadership roles was the confidential mentor they could turn to, who would give them straight talk, and allow them to share what they were going through, without judgment.[2]

The future is always unknown, but that uncertainty cannot be the reason to let mentorship fall by the wayside. It is too valuable an opportunity to lose due to uncertainty or anxiety regarding an unknown outcome.

But we are also realists and recognize that perfect mentorship rarely happens right out of the gate. It takes practice, and several rounds of trial and error. Just because you are successful at what you do does not automatically mean you will be a great mentor. You need the ability to reflect, break things down into small segments, and have endless patience. There are experienced and successful people in every field who are simply not the right fit. Their personality, priorities, bandwidth, or disposition precludes them from serving as an effective mentor to many mentees. Thankfully, those people are the exceptions, not the rule. We believe that by reading this book, you send a strong signal that within you lie the ability, patience, and commitment to learn to become the most effective mentor you can be.

Looking Forward

Globally, there are only a handful of thought leaders on mentorship, and the field is ever evolving. If you'd like to learn more on mentorship in general, or nuances, such as mentoring teams, gender, or mentoring with AI, we have curated some key resources for you in the Appendix. As we know that adults take in and process information differently, we have included resources in various mediums, including books, journals, podcasts, and LinkedIn Learning courses.

We expect the field of mentoring to evolve and be given even greater attention in the years ahead. The reasons are multifaceted. First, the varied roles that a more senior person can have in helping someone more junior—such as traditional mentor, coach, sponsor, connector—have only recently been clearly identified, delineated, and labeled. We expect there will be even more studies and publications about the diversity of mentor types—and how each plays a pivotal role toward a mentee's success. Just as we now have a blueprint for what makes an effective mentor, we will also likely have guidance on what makes an effective coach or a successful sponsor. And we expect a constant evolution of mentoring models that address contextual elements and provide new clarity toward best practice. We are excited about peer mentorship models, virtual mentorship teams, and reverse mentoring, and we look forward to seeing best practices inform these areas.

In 2025, LinkedIn's Workplace Learning Report named mentoring as one of the most effective resources needed to succeed.[3] Those emerging in the field are now prioritizing finding and securing a mentor. Relatedly, departments, institutions, organizations, and companies are focusing on formalizing mentoring relationships by proactively forming mentoring teams or developing "launch" committees. Many organizations have workforce/talent development (or, in higher education, faculty development) leads whose jobs are to ensure that mentoring matches and teams are created and thriving so that mentors and mentees can succeed.

Finally, artificial intelligence is playing an outsized role in mentoring in a way that didn't even exist just a few years ago. While it has its drawbacks, it also has great benefits. Artificial intelligence (AI) is a great enhancer, not a replacement, for mentoring with a human being.[4] Artificial intelligence tools can help identify a mentee's strengths and areas for growth and key domains that could be further developed or strengthened and align these areas with career trajectory. As well, they can scour databases to find individuals who have had similar paths or have deep expertise in specific areas—thus helping facilitate mentor matchmaking. We believe AI and large language models will also play a role in how we think about mentors and the role they play in one's career: an individual who knows their way around AI enhancements to improve workflow could be, for example, a valuable coach for time management. Similarly, sponsors and connectors could use AI-based tools to examine whom they are sponsoring, where, and with what degree of success. Such tools, we believe, will bring a new, data-driven dimension to mentorship that will further enrich and enhance the art.

So what does the future hold? We envision mentoring being top of mind and a strategic priority within healthcare. We are already seeing increased requests for keynotes, workshops, seminars, and teaching sessions on this topic, from medical schools, medical societies, hospitals, and hospital systems. A concerted effort to focus on mentoring through "mentoring academies" will begin to emerge in various academic centers around the globe. The number of qualified executive coaches working within healthcare has skyrocketed over the last decade. In fact, newly appointed senior executives now often negotiate to have an executive coach to guide them throughout their leadership role and often beforehand, when they are negotiating their package. Aligned with this idea, we expect a rise in mentor leaders who will expertly match mentors with mentees and ensure that those relationships are productive and help when they aren't.

An area that deserves extra attention is that of routine evaluations and assessments of how effectively the mentoring pairs or teams are working and how well an organization is prepared to authentically foster and promote mentoring activities. While we often speak to the importance of mentorship, few tools evaluate the quality of how such mentoring is delivered. While we have developed static checklists and have survey-based feedback tools for both individual and programmatic aspects of our mentoring offerings (as in Chapter 14), the field will benefit tremendously from more advanced techniques in this regard. A mentorship quality indicator—that offers input from all members of a mentee's team—can help assess congruence of thoughts/ideas and attribute growth and development more directly to mentorship.

The time is ripe for the more widespread and regular use of organizational mentoring climate surveys that offer a snapshot of how employees within the healthcare system feel about the mentoring that occurs (or doesn't) at their institution. The data generated can be analyzed at the institutional level or at a more granular unit level—can be used to identify problems, highlight areas of opportunity, and develop interventions. When mentoring is inculcated into the organization's culture, such a tool could also be used to recruit mentors and mentees to institutions that score well on such assessments.

We are aware that our views in this book have been US-centric. This is not surprising, given that is where we have been working and mentoring for most of our adult lives. The United States has a robust and well-documented approach to mentoring, as compared with most other countries, including advanced economic nations such as Japan, Australia, India, England, and Italy. This is certainly true for academic medical centers in these countries (which we have been privileged to see firsthand). Therefore, much of the future interest in mentoring development may occur internationally as workforce development and career success are equally important in those countries as it is in the United States.

It is an exciting time to be interested in mentoring. With enormous anticipation, we look forward to both watching and helping shape the future of this important field.

Final Thoughts

We strongly urge you to put aside hesitation and thoughtfully consider being an active participant in a mentorship opportunity. Effective and mutually beneficial mentoring relationships are absolutely critical to career success in every field. Our goal, from the very start of this project, has been that the practical guidance and tools provided throughout the pages of this book help alleviate any trepidations that may have crossed your mind.

Mentors: You have the opportunity to offer real-world experience to emerging members of your field while simultaneously learning more about yourself and your own unique strengths.

Mentees: The right mentor(s) is/are a gold mine of learning and growth experiences that cannot be equated to what you find in a textbook, YouTube video, or TED talk, or via a Google or AI search.

We strongly encourage both mentors and mentees to focus on what could develop—the transformative experience and developing career that could emerge with the right tools and person by your side. With attentive planning and clear communication, well-suited mentors and mentees are poised for a memorable and enjoyable learning adventure that solidifies further growth and success within their field.

Successful mentorship does much more than provide benefits for those involved: It paves the road for further achievement, breakthroughs, and knowledge for generations to come. We hope this book will illuminate your journey. It is a future we look forward to seeing.

Ultimately, when your career fades into memory, it won't be your accomplishments that linger—it's the lives you've touched, guided, and inspired through mentoring that will create your lasting legacy.

Appendix: Additional Resources

Books

Chopra V, Vaughn VM, Saint S. The Mentoring Guide: Helping Mentors and Mentees Succeed. (Suarez, Illus.) Ann Arbor, MI: Michigan Publishing Services; 2019.

Goldsmith M, Reiter M. What Got You Here Won't Get You There: How Successful People Become Even More Successful. New York, NY: Grand Central Publishing; 2007.

Gordon P. Reverse Mentoring: Removing Barriers and Building Belonging in the Workplace. New York, NY: Balance; 2022.

Gotian R, Lopata A. The Financial Times Guide to Mentoring: A Complete Guide to Effective Mentoring (Financial Times Series). Hoboken, NJ: Pearson Education; 2024.

Humphrey HJ. Mentoring in Academic Medicine. Philadelphia, PA: American College of Physicians; 2010.

Johnson WB. On Being a Mentor: A Guide for Higher Education Faculty. 2nd ed. New York, NY: Routledge; 2015.

Johnson WB, Smith DG. Athena Rising: How and Why Men Should Mentor Women. Brighton, MA: Harvard Business Review Press; 2019.

Miller SJ. The Ultimate Guide to Great Mentorship: 13 Roles to Making a True Impact. New York, NY: HarperCollins Leadership; 2023.

Saint S, Chopra V. Thirty Rules for Healthcare Leaders. (Bornstein, Illus.) Ann Arbor, MI: Michigan Publishing Services; 2019.

Starr J. The Mentoring Manual: Your Step-by-Step Guide to Being a Better Mentor. 2nd ed. Hoboken, NJ: Pearson Education; 2021.

Zachary LJ, Fain LZ. The Mentor's Guide: Facilitating Effective Learning Relationships. 3rd ed. Hoboken, NJ: Jossey-Bass; 2022.

LinkedIn Learning Courses

Free with LinkedIn Premium accounts, US library cards, and many enterprise accounts—check if your organization provides complimentary access.

Gordon P. Reverse Mentorship Essentials [online course]: LinkedIn Learning; 2023 [accessed 2025 July 27]. Available from: https://www.linkedin.com/learning/reverse-mentorship-essentials/the-power-of-reverse-mentoring.

Gotian R. Becoming an Inspiring Mentor [online course]: LinkedIn Learning; 2022 [accessed 2025 July 27]. Available from: https://www.linkedin.com/learning/becoming-an-inspiring-mentor/the-business-case-for-mentoring.

Gotian R. Mentoring Employees in the Era of AI [online course]: LinkedIn Learning; 2025 [accessed 2025 July 27]. Available from: https://www.linkedin.com/learning/mentoring-employees-in-the-era-of-ai/why-mentoring-is-more-critical-than-ever.

Gotian R. Mentoring Tips for Senior Leaders [online course]: LinkedIn Learning; 2025 [accessed 2025 July 27]. Available from: https://www.linkedin.com/learning/mentoring-tips-for-senior-leaders/why-being-a-senior-leader-is-crucial-for-this-course.

Online Articles

Chopra V, Dimick J, Saint S. Making Mentorship a Team Effort: Harvard Business Review; 2020 [accessed 2025 July 18]. Available from: https://hbr.org/2020/03/making-mentorship-a-team-effort.

Chopra V, Saint S. 6 Things Every Mentor Should Do: Harvard Business Review; 2017 [accessed 2025 July 18]. Available from: https://hbr.org/2017/03/6-things-every-mentor-should-do.

Chopra V, Saint S. How Doctors Can Be Better Mentors: Harvard Business Review; 2018 [accessed 2025 July 18]. Available from: https://hbr.org/2018/10/how-doctors-can-be-better-mentors.

Chopra V, Saint S. What Mentors Wish Their Mentees Knew: Harvard Business Review; 2017 [accessed 2025 July 18]. Available from: https://hbr.org/2017/11/what-mentors-wish-their-mentees-knew.

Clark D, Redding A. You Don't Need a Mentor to Get the Career Advice You Need: Harvard Business Review; 2025 [accessed 2025 July 18]. Available from: https://hbr.org/2025/03/you-dont-need-a-mentor-to-get-the-career-advice-you-need.

Fessell D, Chopra V, Saint S. Mentoring During a Crisis: Harvard Business Review; 2020 [accessed 2025 July 18]. Available from: https://hbr.org/2020/10/mentoring-during-a-crisis.

Gotian R. Ghosted by Your Mentor? Here's How to Bounce Back Stronger: Psychology Today; 2024 [accessed 2025 July 18]. Available from: https://www.psychologytoday.com/us/blog/optimizing-success/202406/ghosted-by-your-mentor-heres-how-to-bounce-back-stronger.

Gotian R. When a Mentor Dies: Psychology Today; 2024 [accessed 2025 July 18]. Available from: https://www.psychologytoday.com/us/blog/optimizing-success/202402/when-a-mentor-dies.

Gotian R, Lopata A. When the Mentor Feels Like an Imposter: Fast Company; 2025 [accessed 2025 July 18]. Available from: https://www.fastcompany.com/91271347/when-the-mentor-feels-like-an-imposter.

Gotian R, Pfund C, Cook C, Johnson WB. Don't Let Mentoring Burn You Out: Harvard Business Review; 2022 [accessed 2025 July 18]. Available from: https://hbr.org/2022/07/dont-let-mentoring-burn-you-out.

Lachenauer R. What Happens When You Lose Your Mentor: Harvard Business Review; 2019 [accessed 2025 July 18]. Available from: https://hbr.org/2019/06/what-happens-when-you-lose-your-mentor.

Lopata A, Gotian R. Yes, Even CEOs Need Mentors. Here's Why: Fast Company; 2024 [accessed 2025 July 18]. Available from: https://www.fastcompany.com/91138386/yes-even-ceos-need-mentors-heres-why.

Omadeke J. The Importance of Setting Boundaries with Your Mentor: Harvard Business Review; 2024 [accessed 2025 July 18]. Available from: https://hbr.org/2024/06/the-importance-of-setting-boundaries-with-your-mentor.

Why Doctors Make Good Mentors—and 4 Tips to Be Better: Advisory Board; 2018 [accessed 2025 July 18]. Available from: https://www.advisory.com/daily-briefing/2018/11/20/mentor.

Journal Articles

Burgess A, van Diggele C, Mellis C. Mentorship in the Health Professions: A Review. Clin Teach. 2018;15(3):197–202.

Chopra V, Arora VM, Saint S. Will You Be My Mentor?—Four Archetypes to Help Mentees Succeed in Academic Medicine. JAMA Int Med. 2018;178(2):175–6.

Chopra V, Edelson DP, Saint S. Mentorship Malpractice. JAMA. 2016;315(14):1453–4.

Chopra V, Saint S. Mindful Mentorship. Healthc (Amst). 2020;8(1):100390.

Chopra V, Woods MD, Saint S. The Four Golden Rules of Effective Menteeship. BMJ. 2016;354(4147).

Davila JS, Gotian R. Tormentor Mentors, and How to Survive Them. Nature. 2023.

Houchens N, Kuhn L, Ratz D, Su GL, Saint S. Committed to Success: A Structured Mentoring Program for Clinically Oriented Physicians. Mayo Clin Proc Innov Qual Outcomes. 2024;8(4):356–63.

Kuhn L, Saint S, Greene MT, Hayward R, Krein SL. A Group Approach to Clinical Research Mentorship at a Veterans Affairs Medical Center. Fed Pract. 2024;41(11):365–9.

Lee A, Dennis C, Campbell P. Nature's Guide for Mentors. Nature. 2007;447(7146):791–7.

Lefkowitz RJ. Inspiring the Next Generation of Physician-Scientists. J Clin Invest. 2015;125(8):2905–7.

Pfund C, House SC, Asquith P, Fleming MF, Buhr KA, Burnham EL, et al. Training Mentors of Clinical and Translational Research Scholars. Acad Med. 2014;89(5):774–82.

Saint S, Chopra V. Five Questions Every Mentee Should Have an Answer to. Am J Med. 2020;133(7):779–80.

Saint S. Sacred Moments during Mentorship. J Gen Int Med. 2025;40(7):1655–6.

Shoji K, Nishiya K, Miyairi I, Saitoh A, Uematsu S, Ishiguro A, et al. Effective Mentoring in Pediatrics. Pediatr Int. 2023;66(1).

Vaughn V, Saint S, Chopra V. Mentee Missteps: Tales from the Academic Trenches. JAMA. 2017;317(5):475–6.

Waljee JF, Chopra V, Saint S. Mentoring Millennials. JAMA. 2018;319(15):1547–8.

Podcasts

Beard A, Nickisch C. Episode 653: When Men Mentor Women [Internet podcast]: HBR IdeaCast. Harvard Business Review; 2018. Available from: https://podcasts.apple.com/lt/podcast/when-men-mentor-women/id152022135?i=1000422455313.

Chopra V. Michigan Mentoring Podcast [Internet podcast]; 2021. Available from: https://podcasts.apple.com/us/podcast/michigan-mentoring-podcast/id1508379078.

Christian K. Andy Lopata on Mentoring and Relationship Strategies [Internet podcast]: Negotiate Anything. American Negotiation Institute; 2024. Available from: https://open.spotify.com/episode/6JaZ99NYb7frNxOYol4xj4.

Gupta A. The Art and Science of Choosing a Mentor with Dr. Sanjay Saint [Internet podcast]: The Medicine Mentors Podcast. 2020. Available from: https://open.spotify.com/episode/4TwBRznaEEZyb6X5R9k9pi.

Gupta A. The Medicine Mentors Podcast [Internet podcast]; 2025. Available from: https://open.spotify.com/show/28UQu1hWWvU3wucTwo4Lvc.

Lopata A. Connected Leadership Gold: Mentoring with Vanessa Vallely and Kerrie Dorman [Internet podcast]: The Connected Leadership Podcast. Evergreen Podcasts; 2023. Available from: https://podfollow.com/connectedleadership/episode/8f2afeac76fc2dc563d95a3f41c2ac1e0b352dc8/view.

Lopata A. Episode 222: Leading in the NHS with Tendai Wileman [Internet podcast]: The Connected Leadership Podcast. Evergreen Podcasts; 2024. Available from: https://podfollow.com/connectedleadership/episode/03097a54d592ea0a4f9d42036da97fd9dc3692e0/view.

Stachowiak D. Episode 684: How to Be a Better Mentor, with Ruth Gotian [Internet podcast]: Coaching for Leaders. Innovate Learning; 2024. Available from: https://open.spotify.com/episode/5qzcrvTlbQkHvrjiTafwoC?si=NqslEugJRISqtj7mIJtKpg&nd=1&dlsi=f0efc0c596c44f6f.

Talks

Gordon P. Reverse Mentorship: When Leaders Listen to their Employees [video]: TEDx Talks; 2024 [accessed 2025 July 18]. Available from: https://www.youtube.com/watch?v=44-MDhdbn1E.

Harris C. How to Find the Person Who Can Help You Get Ahead at Work [video]: TED talks; 2018 [accessed 2025 July 27]. Available from: https://www.ted.com/talks/carla_harris_how_to_find_the_person_who_can_help_you_get_ahead_at_work.

University of Colorado Department of Medicine. Mentorship Academy 2023 [video] YouTube; 2023 [accessed 2025 July 18]. Available from: https://www.youtube.com/watch?v=pTYMeo6biOE.

Other

Center for the Improvement of Mentored Experiences in Research [accessed 2025 July 18]. Available from: https://cimerproject.org/.

Gotian R. Developing Your Mentoring Team: A Workbook; 2024 [accessed 2025 July 18]. Available from: https://ruthgotian.com/mentoringteam/.

International Mentoring Association [accessed 2025 July 18]. Available from: https://www.mentoringassociation.org/.

National Academies of Sciences, Engineering, and Medicine; Policy and Global Affairs; Board on Higher Education and Workforce; Committee on Effective Mentoring in STEMM; Byars Winston-A, Dahlberg ML. *The Science of Effective Mentorship in STEMM.* Washington, DC: National Academies Press (US); 2019.

References

Chapter 1. Three Steps to Getting Started as a Mentor

1. Gawande A. The Checklist Manifesto: How to Get Things Right. New York, NY: Metropolitan Books; 2011.
2. Chopra V, Dimick J, Saint S. Making Mentorship a Team Effort: Harvard Business Review; 2020 [accessed 2025 July 18]. Available from: https://hbr.org/2020/03/making-mentorship-a-team-effort.
3. Chopra V, Edelson DP, Saint S. Mentorship Malpractice. JAMA. 2016;315(14): 1453–4.
4. Gardner WL, Martinko MJ. Using the Myers-Briggs Type Indicator to Study Managers: A Literature Review and Research Agenda. J Manag. 1996;22(1):45–83.
5. Comaford C. 76% of People Think Mentors Are Important, But Only 37% Have One: Forbes; 2019 [accessed 2025 July 22]. Available from: https://www.forbes.com/sites/christinecomaford/2019/07/03/new-study-76-of-people-think-mentors-are-important-but-only-37-have-one/.
6. Vaughn V, Saint S, Chopra V. Mentee Missteps: Tales from the Academic Trenches. JAMA. 2017;317(5):475–6.

Chapter 2. Know Your Role

1. Chopra V, Arora VM, Saint S. Will You Be My Mentor?—Four Archetypes to Help Mentees Succeed in Academic Medicine. JAMA Int Med. 2018;178(2):175–6.
2. Claman P. Forget Mentors: Employ a Personal Board of Directors: Harvard Business Review; 2010 [accessed 2025 July 22]. Available from: https://hbr.org/2010/10/forget-mentors-employ-a-person.
3. Gordon P. Reverse Mentoring: Removing Barriers and Building Belonging in the Workplace. New York, NY: Balance; 2022.
4. Moniz MH, Saint S. Leadership & Professional Development: Be the Change You Want to See. J Hosp Med. 2019;14(4):254.
5. Gawande A. Personal Best: The New Yorker; 2011 [accessed 2025 July 22]. Available from: https://www.newyorker.com/magazine/2011/10/03/personal-best.

6. Houchens N, Harrod M, Saint S. Teaching Inpatient Medicine: Connecting, Coaching, and Communicating in the Hospital. 2nd ed. New York, NY: Oxford University Press; 2023.

7. Kuhn L, Saint S, Greene MT, Hayward R, Krein SL. A Group Approach to Clinical Research Mentorship at a Veterans Affairs Medical Center. Fed Pract. 2024;41(11):365–9.

8. Richardson J, Postmes T, Stroebe K. Social Capital, Identification and Support: Scope for Integration. PLoS One. 2022;17(4).

9. Ibarra H. How to Do Sponsorship Right: Harvard Business Review; 2022 [accessed 2024 July 22]. Available from: https://hbr.org/2022/11/how-to-do-sponsorship-right.

10. Women in the Workplace: McKinsey & Company; 2016 [accessed 2025 August 1]. Available from: https://www.mckinsey.com/featured-insights/diversity-and-inclusion/women-in-the-workplace-archive#section-header-2016.

11. Thomas DA. Race Matters: Harvard Business Review; 2001 [accessed 2024 July 22]. Available from: https://hbr.org/2001/04/race-matters.

12. Schwartz R, Williams MF, Feldman MD. Does Sponsorship Promote Equity in Career Advancement in Academic Medicine? A Scoping Review. J Gen Int Med. 2023;39(3):470–80.

13. Ibarra H, Carter NM, Silva C. Why Men Still Get More Promotions Than Women: Harvard Business Review; 2010 [accessed 2025 July 22]. Available from: https://hbr.org/2010/09/why-men-still-get-more-promotions-than-women.

14. McPherson M, Smith-Lovin L, Cook JM. Birds of a Feather: Homophily in Social Networks. Ann Rev Sociol. 2001;27(1):415–44.

15. Gladwell M. The Tipping Point: How Little Things Can Make a Big Difference. New York, NY: Back Bay Books; 2002.

16. Clark D. Joining a Professional Group Where Everyone Already Knows Each Other: Harvard Business Review; 2024 [accessed 2025 July 22]. Available from: https://hbr.org/2024/12/joining-a-professional-group-where-everyone-already-knows-each-other.

Chapter 3. Six Rules for Effective Mentoring

1. Gotian R. Why Your Boss Shouldn't Be Your Mentor: Forbes; 2020 [accessed 2025 July 22]. Available from: https://www.forbes.com/sites/ruthgotian/2020/10/16/why-your-boss-shouldnt-be-your-mentor/.

2. Gross CJ. A Better Approach to Mentorship: Harvard Business Review; 2023 [accessed 2025 July 25]. Available from: https://hbr.org/2023/06/a-better-approach-to-mentorship.

3. Chopra V, Edelson DP, Saint S. Mentorship Malpractice. JAMA. 2016;315(14): 1453–4.

4. Weller J, Gotian R. Evolution of the Feedback Conversation in Anaesthesia Education: A Narrative Review. Br J Anaesth. 2023;131(3):503–9.

5. Chopra V, Saint S. How Doctors Can Be Better Mentors: Harvard Business Review; 2018 [accessed 2025 July 18]. Available from: https://hbr.org/2018/10/how-doctors-can-be-better-mentors.

6. Parkinson's Law: The Economist; 1955 [Archive] [accessed 2025 July 18]. Available from: https://web.archive.org/web/20180705215319/https://www.economist.com/news/1955/11/19/parkinsons-law.

Chapter 4. Mentorship Malpractice: From Mentor to Tormentor

1. Woolston C. A Message for Mentors from Dissatisfied Graduate Students. Nature. 2019;575(7783):551–2.
2. Woolston C. Stress and Uncertainty Drag down Graduate Students' Satisfaction. Nature. 2022;610(7933):805–8.
3. National Academies of Sciences, Engineering, and Medicine; Policy and Global Affairs; Board on Higher Education and Workforce; Committee on Effective Mentoring in STEMM; Byars Winston-A, Dahlberg ML. The Science of Effective Mentorship in STEMM. Washington, DC: National Academies Press (US); 2019.
4. Davila JS, Gotian R. Tormentor Mentors, and How to Survive Them. Nature. 2023.
5. Chopra V, Edelson DP, Saint S. Mentorship Malpractice. JAMA. 2016;315(14): 1453–4.
6. Gotian R, Pfund C, Cook C, Johnson WB. Don't Let Mentoring Burn You Out: Harvard Business Review; 2022 [accessed 2025 July 18]. Available from: https://hbr.org/2022/07/dont-let-mentoring-burn-you-out.
7. Chen C, Liao J, Wen P. Why Does Formal Mentoring Matter? The Mediating Role of Psychological Safety and the Moderating Role of Power Distance Orientation in the Chinese Context. Int J Hum Resour Manag. 2014;25(8):1112–30.
8. Scandura TA. Dysfunctional Mentoring Relationships and Outcomes. J Manag. 1998;24(3):449–67.
9. Eby LT, Allen TD, Evans SC, Ng T, Dubois D. Does Mentoring Matter? A Multidisciplinary Meta-Analysis Comparing Mentored and Non-Mentored Individuals. J Vocat Behav. 2008;72(2):254–67.
10. Allen TD, Eby LT, Poteet ML, Lentz E, Lima L. Career Benefits Associated with Mentoring for Proteges: A Meta-Analysis. J Appl Psychol. 2004;89(1): 127–36.
11. Eby LT, Allen TD. Further Investigation of Protégés' Negative Mentoring Experiences. Group Organ Manag. 2002;27(4):456–79.
12. Ragins BR, Cotton JL, Miller JS. Marginal Mentoring: The Effects of Type of Mentor, Quality of Relationship, and Program Design on Work and Career Attitudes. Acad Manag J. 2000;43(6):1177–94.
13. Workplace Loyalties Change, But the Value of Mentoring Doesn't [Internet podcast]: Knowledge at Wharton Podcast. The Wharton School of the University of Pennsylvania; 2007. Available from: https://knowledge.wharton.upenn.edu/podcast/knowledge-at-wharton-podcast/workplace-loyalties-change-but-the-value-of-mentoring-doesnt/.
14. Carucci RA. To Be Honest: Lead with the Power of Truth, Justice and Purpose. New York, NY: Kogan Page; 2021.
15. Shanafelt TD, Gorringe G, Menaker R, Storz KA, Reeves D, Buskirk SJ, et al. Impact of Organizational Leadership on Physician Burnout and Satisfaction. Mayo Clin Proc. 2015;90(4):432–40.
16. Housman M, Minor D. Organizational Design and Space: The Good, the Bad, and the Productive: Harvard Business School Working Papers; 2016 [accessed 2025 July 25]. Available from: https://doi.org/10.2139/ssrn.2805578.

Chapter 5. Mentoring across Differences

1. Viglione G. Chemists Grapple with Lack of Diversity Displayed in "Dude Walls" of Honor: Chemical & Engineering News; 2019 [accessed 2025 July 22]. Available from: https://cen.acs.org/careers/diversity/Chemists-grapple-lack-diversity-displayed/97/i37.

2. Boyle P. More Women Than Men Are Enrolled in Medical School: AAMC; 2019 [accessed 2025 July 18]. Available from: https://www.aamc.org/news/more-women-men-are-enrolled-medical-school.

3. Byrne DE. The Attraction Paradigm. New York, NY: Academic Press; 1971.

4. Montoya RM, Horton RS, Kirchner J. Is Actual Similarity Necessary for Attraction? A Meta-Analysis of Actual and Perceived Similarity. J Soc Pers Relat. 2008;25(6):889–922.

5. Page SE. The Difference: How the Power of Diversity Creates Better Groups, Firms, Schools, and Societies. Princeton, NJ: Princeton University Press; 2008.

6. Phillips KW. How Diversity Makes Us Smarter: Scientific American; 2014 [accessed 2025 July 18]. Available from: https://www.scientificamerican.com/article/how-diversity-makes-us-smarter/.

7. Rock D, Grant H. Why Diverse Teams Are Smarter: Harvard Business Review; 2016 [accessed 2025 July 22]. Available from: https://hbr.org/2016/11/why-diverse-teams-are-smarter.

8. Tversky A, Kahneman D. Judgment under Uncertainty: Heuristics and Biases. Science. 1974;185(4157):1124–31.

9. Moniz MH, Saint S. Leadership & Professional Development: Be the Change You Want to See. J Hosp Med. 2019;14(4):254.

10. Collier KM, James CA, Saint S, Howell JD. The Role of Spirituality and Religion in Physician and Trainee Wellness. J Gen Int Med. 2021;36(10):3199–201.

11. Collier KM, James CA, Saint S, Howell JD. Is It Time to More Fully Address Teaching Religion and Spirituality in Medicine? Ann Intern Med. 2020;172(12):817–8.

12. Collier KM, Greene MT, Ratz D, Ehrlinger R, Saint S. Spirituality and Religiosity of Internal Medicine Physicians in the USA: Results from a National Survey. J Gen Int Med. 2025 [online ahead of print].

13. Gilligan C. In a Different Voice: Psychological Theory and Women's Development. Cambridge, MA: Harvard University Press; 2016.

14. Helgesen S, Goldsmith M. How Women Rise: Break the 12 Habits Holding You Back from Your Next Raise, Promotion, or Job. New York, NY: Hachette Books; 2018.

15. Ibarra H, Carter NM, Silva C. Why Men Still Get More Promotions Than Women: Harvard Business Review; 2010 [accessed 2025 July 22]. Available from: https://hbr.org/2010/09/why-men-still-get-more-promotions-than-women.

16. Johnson B, Smith D, Gotian R. Note to Men: Mentor Her! (Yes, Even during a Pandemic): Chief Learning Officer; 2020 [accessed 2025 July 18]. Available from: https://www.chieflearningofficer.com/2020/07/14/note-to-men-mentor-her-yes-even-during-a-pandemic/.

17. Johnson WB, Smith DG. Athena Rising: How and Why Men Should Mentor Women. Brighton, MA: Harvard Business Review Press; 2019.

18. Jain S, Gotian R. When You Recommend Someone for an Opportunity, Follow through. Nature. 2021.

19. Mody L, Howell JD, Saint S. Success in Science: What We Can Learn from Women Artists. J Clin Invest. 2019;129(11):4560–2.

20. Gotian R, Lopata A. The Financial Times Guide to Mentoring: A Complete Guide to Effective Mentoring (Financial Times Series). Hoboken, NJ: Pearson Education; 2024.

21. Lawrence C, Mhlaba T, Stewart KA, Moletsane R, Gaede B, Moshabela M. The Hidden Curricula of Medical Education: A Scoping Review. Acad Med. 2018;93(4):648–56.

22. Levine RB, Ayyala MS, Skarupski KA, Bodurtha JN, Fernandez MG, Ishii LE, et al. "It's a Little Different for Men"—Sponsorship and Gender in Academic Medicine: A Qualitative Study. J Gen Intern Med. 2021;36(1):1–8.

23. Schwartz R, Williams MF, Feldman MD. Does Sponsorship Promote Equity in Career Advancement in Academic Medicine? A Scoping Review. J Gen Int Med. 2023;39(3):470–80.

24. Nancekivell SE, Shah P, Gelman SA. Maybe They're Born with It, or Maybe It's Experience: Toward a Deeper Understanding of the Learning Style Myth. J Educ Psychol. 2020;112(2):221–35.

25. Kolb D. Learning Style Inventory: Self Scoring Test and Interpretation Booklet. Boston, MA: McBer & Company; 1985.

26. Drago-Severson E. Leading Adult Learning: Supporting Adult Development in Our Schools. Thousand Oaks, CA: Corwin; 2009.

27. Edmondson A. Psychological Safety and Learning Behavior in Work Teams. Adm Sci Q. 1999;44(2):350–83.

28. Gotian R. This Is Why High Performers Crave Feedback: Fast Company; 2025 [accessed 2025 July 22]. Available from: https://www.fastcompany.com/91277346/this-is-why-high-performers-crave-feedback.

29. Gotian R. Networking for Introverted Scientists. Nature. 2019.

30. Gotian R. Why You Earned the Right to Have Imposter Syndrome: Psychology Today; 2021 [accessed 2025 July 22]. Available from: https://www.psychology-today.com/us/blog/optimizing-success/202104/why-you-earned-the-right-to-have-imposter-syndrome.

31. Chopra V, Greene MT, Engle JM, Fowler KE, Saint S. Mentorship in General Internal Medicine: Results from a National Survey. J Gen Int Med. 2025 [online ahead of print].

Chapter 6. Mentoring in a Virtual Era

1. Accreditation Council for Graduate Medical Education (ACGME). The ACGME's Approach to Limit Resident Duty Hours 12 Months after Implementation: A Summary of Achievements. 2004.

2. Gotian R. How Do You Find a Decent Mentor When You're Stuck at Home?: Harvard Business Review; 2020 [accessed 2025 July 23]. Available from: https://hbr.org/2020/08/how-do-you-find-a-decent-mentor-when-youre-stuck-at-home.

3. Pursell H. How to Use AI Tools for Coaching and Mentoring: Guider; 2023 [accessed 2025 July 25]. Available from: https://guider-ai.com/blog/ai-for-mentoring-and-coaching/.

4. Edmondson A. Psychological Safety and Learning Behavior in Work Teams. Adm Sci Q. 1999;44(2):350–83.

5. Weller J, Gotian R. Evolution of the Feedback Conversation in Anaesthesia Education: A Narrative Review. Br J Anaesth. 2023;131(3):503–9.

Chapter 7. The Mentee's Quick-Start Guide

1. Saint S, Chopra V. Chapter 2: Forge the Followers You Want. In: Thirty Rules for Healthcare Leaders. (Bornstein, Illus.) Ann Arbor, MI: Michigan Publishing Services; 2019. p. 9–12.
2. Cho CS, Ramanan RA, Feldman MD. Defining the Ideal Qualities of Mentorship: A Qualitative Analysis of the Characteristics of Outstanding Mentors. Am J Med. 2011;124(5):453–8.
3. Fleming M, Burnham EL, Huskins WC. Mentoring Translational Science Investigators. JAMA. 2012;308(19):1981–2.
4. Stamm M, Buddeberg-Fischer B. The Impact of Mentoring during Postgraduate Training on Doctors' Career Success. Med Educ. 2011;45(5):488–96.
5. Johnson WB. The Intentional Mentor: Strategies and Guidelines for the Practice of Mentoring. Prof Psychol Res Pr. 2002;33(1):88–96.
6. Chopra V, Woods MD, Saint S. The Four Golden Rules of Effective Menteeship. BMJ. 2016;354(4147).
7. Chopra V, Arora VM, Saint S. Will You Be My Mentor?—Four Archetypes to Help Mentees Succeed in Academic Medicine. JAMA Int Med. 2018;178(2):175–6.
8. Saint S, Chopra V. Five Questions Every Mentee Should Have an Answer to. Am J Med. 2020;133(7):779–80.
9. Gotian R. How to Find the Perfect Mentor to Boost Your Career: Forbes; 2021 [accessed 2025 July 23]. Available from: https://www.forbes.com/sites/ruthgotian/2021/01/26/how-to-find-the-perfect-mentor-to-boost-your-career/.

Chapter 8. Nine Things Standout Mentees Do

1. Goldsmith M, Reiter M. What Got You Here Won't Get You There: How Successful People become Even More Successful. New York, NY: Grand Central Publishing; 2007.
2. Saint S, Chopra V. Chapter 5: Beef up Your EQ. In: Thirty Rules for Healthcare Leaders. (Bornstein, Illus.) Ann Arbor, MI: Michigan Publishing Services; 2019. p. 21–4.
3. Lyons M. 5 Essential Soft Skills to Develop in Any Job: Harvard Business Review; 2023 [accessed 2025 July 23]. Available from: https://hbr.org/2023/02/5-essential-soft-skills-to-develop-in-any-job.
4. Gladwell M. Blink: The Power of Thinking without Thinking. New York, NY: Back Bay Books; 2007.
5. Bandura A. Social Learning Theory. Englewood Cliffs, NJ: Prentice-Hall; 1976.
6. Passi V, Johnson S, Peile E, Wright S, Hafferty F, Johnson N. Doctor Role Modelling in Medical Education: BEME Guide No. 27. Med Teach. 2013;35(9):e1422–36.
7. Baldwin A, Mills J, Birks M, Budden L. Role Modeling in Undergraduate Nursing Education: An Integrative Literature Review. Nurse Educ Today. 2014;34(6):e18–26.
8. Lopata A, Gotian R. Yes, Even CEOs Need Mentors. Here's Why: Fast Company; 2024 [accessed 2025 July 18]. Available from: https://www.fastcompany.com/91138386/yes-even-ceos-need-mentors-heres-why.
9. Saint S. Sacred Moments during Mentorship. J Gen Int Med. 2025;40(7):1655–6.

10. Chopra V, Saint S. What Mentors Wish Their Mentees Knew: Harvard Business Review; 2017 [accessed 2025 July 18]. Available from: https://hbr.org/2017/11/what-mentors-wish-their-mentees-knew.
11. Dweck CS. Mindset: The New Psychology of Success. New York, NY: Ballantine Books; 2007.
12. Saint S, Chopra V. Chapter 4: Watch Your TLR. In: Thirty Rules for Healthcare Leaders. (Bornstein, Illus.) Ann Arbor, MI: Michigan Publishing Services; 2019. p. 17–20.
13. This is Why Senior Executives Stop Hearing the Truth. Fast Company, 2025. [Accessed October 17, 2025]. Available from https://www.fastcompany.com/91394613/this-is-why-senior-executives-stop-hearing-the-truth.

Chapter 9. Beware of the Mentee Landmines

1. Edmondson AC. Right Kind of Wrong: The Science of Failing Well. New York, NY: Simon Element/Simon Acumen; 2023.
2. Vaughn V, Saint S, Chopra V. Mentee Missteps: Tales from the Academic Trenches. JAMA. 2017;317(5):475–6.
3. Ury W. The Power of a Positive No: How to Say No and Still Get to Yes. New York, NY: Bantam Books; 2007.
4. Edmondson AC. The Fearless Organization: Creating Psychological Safety in the Workplace for Learning, Innovation, and Growth. Hoboken, NJ: John Wiley & Sons, Inc; 2019.

Chapter 10. Moving On from a Mentoring Relationship: Knowing When It's Time

1. Houchens N, Kuhn L, Ratz D, Su GL, Saint S. Committed to Success: A Structured Mentoring Program for Clinically Oriented Physicians. Mayo Clin Proc Innov Qual Outcomes. 2024;8(4):356–63.

Chapter 11. Menteeship for Clinicians and Non-Researchers

1. Saint S, Chopra V. Five Questions Every Mentee Should Have an Answer to. Am J Med. 2020;133(7):779–80.
2. Gotian R. The Success Factor: Developing the Mindset and Skillset for Peak Business Performance. London, UK: Kogan Page; 2022.
3. University of Colorado Department of Medicine. Mentorship Academy: The Regents of the University of Colorado; 2025 [accessed 2025 July 23]. Available from: https://medschool.cuanschutz.edu/medicine/calendar/mentorshipacademy.
4. University of Colorado Department of Medicine. Department of Medicine Mentoring Program: The Regents of the University of Colorado; 2025 [accessed 2025 July 23]. Available from: https://medschool.cuanschutz.edu/medicine/faculty-and-staff-affairs/mentorship/faculty-mentorship.

5. Ragins BR, Cotton JL. Mentor Functions and Outcomes: A Comparison of Men and Women in Formal and Informal Mentoring Relationships. J Appl Psychol. 1999;84(4):529–50.
6. Chao GT, Walz P, Gardner PD. Formal and Informal Mentorships: A Comparison on Mentoring Functions and Contrast with Nonmentored Counterparts. Pers Psychol. 2006;45(3):619–36.
7. Ragins BR, Cotton JL. Easier Said Than Done: Gender Differences in Perceived Barriers to Gaining a Mentor. Acad Manag J. 1991;34(4):939–51.
8. Lopata A. Connected Leadership: How Professional Relationships Underpin Executive Success. St Albans, UK: Panoma Press; 2020.
9. Gotian R, Camarda CJ, Turnbull ZA. What Space Exploration and Health Care Can Teach You about Navigating Uncertainty: Harvard Business Review; 2024 [accessed 2025 July 18]. Available from: https://hbr.org/2024/04/what-space-exploration-and-health-care-can-teach-you-about-navigating-uncertainty.

Chapter 12. Mentoring across Generations: Find Your Common Ground

1. Twenge JM, Campbell WK, Freeman EC. Generational Differences in Young Adults' Life Goals, Concern for Others, and Civic Orientation, 1966–2009. J Pers Soc Psychol. 2012;102(5):1045–62.
2. Huyler D, Gomez L, Rocco TS, Plakhotnik MS. Leading Different Generational Cohorts in the Workplace: Focus on Situational and Inclusive Leadership. New Horiz Adult Educ. 2024;37(1):6–19.
3. Waljee JF, Chopra V, Saint S. Mentoring Millennials. JAMA. 2018;319(15): 1547–8.
4. Pollak L. The Remix: How to Lead and Succeed in the Multigenerational Workplace. New York, NY: Harper Business; 2019.
5. Kolb AY, Kolb DA. Learning Styles and Learning Spaces: Enhancing Experiential Learning in Higher Education. Acad Manage Learn Educ. 2005;4(2):193–212.
6. Kolb DA. Experiential Learning: Experience as the Source of Learning and Development. Englewood Cliffs, NJ: Prentice-Hall; 1984.
7. Siegel B. Building Effective Mentorship Programs for Gen-Z Employees: Forbes; 2023 [accessed 2025 July 24]. Available from: https://www.forbes.com/councils/forbesbusinesscouncil/2023/09/05/building-effective-mentorship-programs-for-gen-z-employees/.
8. Ensher EA, Johnson WB, Smith DG. How to Mentor in a Remote Workplace: Harvard Business Review; 2022 [accessed 2025 July 24]. Available from: https://hbr.org/2022/03/how-to-mentor-in-a-remote-workplace.

Chapter 13. Mentorship and Leadership: Where Paths Converge

1. Cook C, Lopata A, Gotian R. Your Company Needs to Pay Attention to Mentorship. Here's Why: Fast Company; 2024 [accessed 2025 July 24]. Available from: https://www.fastcompany.com/91127022/your-company-needs-to-pay-attention-to-mentorship-heres-why.

2. Smith TM. First Physician Job Post-Residency Often a Way Station: Survey: American Medical Association; 2024 [accessed 2025 July 24]. Available from: https://www.ama-assn.org/medical-residents/transition-resident-attending/first-physician-job-post-residency-often-way.

3. Stamy CD, Schwartz CC, Han LP, Schwinn DA. Community and Academic Physicians Working Together in Integrated Health Care Systems. Mayo Clin Proc Innov Qual Outcomes. 2021;5(5):951–60.

4. Mallon WT, Cox N. Promotion and Tenure Policies and Practices at U.S. Medical Schools: Is Tenure Irrelevant or More Relevant Than Ever? Acad Med. 2024;99(7):724–32.

5. Gotian R, Lopata A. The Financial Times Guide to Mentoring: A Complete Guide to Effective Mentoring (Financial Times Series). Hoboken, NJ: Pearson Education; 2024.

6. Edelman Trust Barometer [accessed 2025 July 24]. Available from: https://www.edelman.com/trust/trust-barometer.

7. Edelman Trust Barometer: Special Report, Trust in the Workplace: Edelman; 2022 [accessed 2025 July 24]. Available from: https://www.edelman.com/sites/g/files/aatuss191/files/2022-08/2022%20Edelman%20Trust%20Barometer%20Special%20Report%20Trust%20in%20the%20Workplace%20FINAL.pdf.

8. Carucci RA. To Be Honest: Lead with the Power of Truth, Justice and Purpose. New York, NY: Kogan Page; 2021.

9. Edmondson A. Psychological Safety and Learning Behavior in Work Teams. Adm Sci Q. 1999;44(2):350–83.

10. Warren R. The Purpose Driven Life: What on Earth Am I Here for? Grand Rapids, MI: Zondervan; 2013.

11. Cameron K. Positively Energizing Leadership: Virtuous Actions and Relationships That Create High Performance. Oakland, CA: Berrett-Koehler Publishers; 2021.

12. Saint S, Chopra V. Chapter 30: Lead with Kindness, Compassion and Love. In: Thirty Rules for Healthcare Leaders. (Bornstein, Illus.) Ann Arbor, MI: Michigan Publishing Services; 2019. p. 121–3.

13. Knowles M. Self-Directed Learning: A Guide for Learners and Teachers. New York, NY: Association Press; 1975.

14. Kolb DA. Experiential Learning: Experience as the Source of Learning and Development. Englewood Cliffs, NJ: Prentice-Hall; 1984.

15. Mezirow J. Transformative Dimensions of Adult Learning. San Francisco, CA: Jossey-Bass; 1991.

16. Saint S. Sacred Moments during Mentorship. J Gen Int Med. 2025;40(7):1655–6.

Chapter 14. Evaluating Mentoring Programs

1. Drucker PF. The Practice of Management. New York, NY: Harper & Row; 1954.

2. Brookfield S. Critically Reflective Practice. J Contin Educ Health Prof. 1998;18(4):197–205.

3. Vosshall L. Anonymous Lab Survey [Survey]; 2019 [accessed 2025 July 24]. Available from: https://docs.google.com/forms/d/e/1FAIpQLScGCi7iACgmVBhFcE7G90oPwuTs-g9CQkrDmOUoQ4FvoT9CfA/viewform.

4. Vosshall L (@leslievosshall). Think Your Lab Is Happy?—Ask Them!! Anonymous Lab Survey [Survey link]: Twitter; February 7, 2022 [accessed 2025 July 24]. Available from: https://x.com/leslievosshall/status/1490841524623769600.

5. Turner ME, Pratkanis AR. Twenty-Five Years of Groupthink Theory and Research: Lessons from the Evaluation of a Theory. Organ Behav Hum Decis Process. 1998;73(2–3):105–15.

6. Schuessler JB, Wilder B, Byrd LW. Reflective Journaling and Development of Cultural Humility in Students. Nurs Educ Perspect. 2012;33(2):96–9.

7. Cranton P. Understanding and Promoting Transformative Learning: A Guide to Theory and Practice. 3rd ed. New York, NY: Routledge; 2016.

8. Tendler BC, Welland M, Miller KL. Why Every Lab Needs a Handbook: eLife; 2023 [accessed 2025 July 24]. Available from: https://elifesciences.org/articles/88853.

9. Hafferty FW. Beyond Curriculum Reform: Confronting Medicine's Hidden Curriculum. Acad Med. 1998;73(4):403–7.

10. Chew LD, Watanabe JM, Buchwald D, Lessler DS. Junior Faculty's Perspectives on Mentoring. Acad Med. 2003;78(6).

11. Houchens N, Kuhn L, Ratz D, Su GL, Saint S. Committed to Success: A Structured Mentoring Program for Clinically Oriented Physicians. Mayo Clin Proc Innov Qual Outcomes. 2024;8(4):356–63.

12. Chopra V, Dimick J, Saint S. Making Mentorship a Team Effort: Harvard Business Review; 2020 [accessed 2025 July 18]. Available from: https://hbr.org/2020/03/making-mentorship-a-team-effort.

13. Kuhn L, Saint S, Greene MT, Hayward R, Krein SL. A Group Approach to Clinical Research Mentorship at a Veterans Affairs Medical Center. Fed Pract. 2024;41(11):365–9.

Chapter 15. Mindfulness in the Mentorship Relationship

1. Pargament KI, Lomax JW, McGee JS, Fang Q. Sacred Moments in Psychotherapy from the Perspectives of Mental Health Providers and Clients: Prevalence, Predictors, and Consequences. Spiritual Clin Pract (Wash DC). 2014;1(4):248–62.

2. Gilmartin H, Saint S, Rogers M, Winter S, Snyder A, Quinn M, et al. Pilot Randomised Controlled Trial to Improve Hand Hygiene through Mindful Moments. BMJ Qual Saf. 2018;27(10):799–806.

3. Chopra V, Saint S. Mindful Mentorship. Healthc (Amst). 2020;8(1):100390.

4. Niemiec RM. The Heartful Way: Mindfulness, Then Heartfulness: Psychology Today; 2015 [accessed 2025 July 24]. Available from: https://www.psychologytoday.com/us/blog/what-matters-most/201510/the-heartful-way-mindfulness-then-heartfulness.

5. Gilmartin HM, Saint S. Finding Joy in Medicine: A Remedy for Challenging Times. NEJM Catalyst. 2022;3(5).

6. Chopra V, Edelson DP, Saint S. Mentorship Malpractice. JAMA. 2016; 315(14):1453–4.

7. Vaughn V, Saint S, Chopra V. Mentee Missteps: Tales from the Academic Trenches. JAMA. 2017;317(5):475–6.

8. Gotian R. 10 Easy Ways to Elevate Your Active Listening Skills: Psychology Today; 2023 [accessed 2025 July 24]. Available from: https://www.psychologytoday.

com/us/blog/optimizing-success/202305/10-easy-ways-to-elevate-your-active-listening-skills.

9. Houchens N, Harrod M, Moody S, Fowler KE, Saint S. Techniques and Behaviors Associated with Exemplary Inpatient General Medicine Teaching: An Exploratory Qualitative Study. J Hosp Med. 2017;12(7):503–9.

10. Saint S, Bloor L, Chopra V. Motivational Interviewing for Healthcare Providers: The BMJ Opinion; 2016 [accessed 2025 July 24]. Available from: https://blogs.bmj.com/bmj/2016/11/30/vineet-chopra-et-al-motivational-interviewing-for-healthcare-providers/.

11. Miller WR, Rollnick S. Motivational Interviewing: Preparing People for Change. 2nd ed. New York, NY: The Guilford Press; 2002.

12. Edmondson AC. The Fearless Organization: Creating Psychological Safety in the Workplace for Learning, Innovation, and Growth. Hoboken, NJ: John Wiley & Sons, Inc; 2019.

13. Bandura A. Self-Efficacy: Toward a Unifying Theory of Behavioral Change. Psychol Rev. 1977;84(2):191–215.

14. Griffith FJ, Wong S, Dietrich KM, Exline JJ, Pargament KI. "The Music Was Speaking to Me": Using Narrative Inquiry to Describe Sacred Moments with Music. Arts Psychother. 2022;79:101911.

15. Quinn M, Fowler KE, Harrod M, Ehrlinger R, Engle JM, Houchens N, et al. Exploring Sacred Moments in Hospitalized Patients: An Exploratory Qualitative Study. J Gen Int Med. 2023;38(9):2038–44.

16. Saint K, Ehrlinger R, Gilliland J, Barton MF, Xu AJ, Santos PMG, et al. A Qualitative Exploration of Sacred Moments in Radiation Oncology. Adv Radiat Oncol. 2024;9(11):101617.

17. Saint S. Sacred Moments during Mentorship. J Gen Int Med. 2025;40(7):1655–6.

18. Koven S. What Is a Mentor? N Engl J Med. 2024;390(8):683–5.

Chapter 16. Looking Back While Traveling Forward

1. Gotian R. How to Find the Perfect Mentor to Boost Your Career: Forbes; 2021 [accessed 2025 July 23]. Available from: https://www.forbes.com/sites/ruthgotian/2021/01/26/how-to-find-the-perfect-mentor-to-boost-your-career/.

2. Lopata A, Gotian R. Yes, Even CEOs Need Mentors. Here's Why: Fast Company; 2024 [accessed 2025 July 18]. Available from: https://www.fastcompany.com/91138386/yes-even-ceos-need-mentors-heres-why.

3. Workplace Learning Report: The Rise of Career Champions: LinkedIn; 2025 [accessed 2025 July 24]. Available from: https://learning.linkedin.com/content/dam/me/learning/en-us/images/lls-workplace-learning-report/2025/full-page/pdfs/LinkedIn-Workplace-Learning-Report-2025.pdf.

4. Lopata A, Gotian R. This Is How AI Is Changing Mentorship: Fast Company; 2025 [accessed 2025 July 24]. Available from: https://www.fastcompany.com/91325756/this-is-how-ai-is-changing-mentorship.

Index

Note: Page numbers in *italics* indicate a figure and page numbers in **bold** indicate a table, box, or worksheet on the corresponding page.

For Product Safety Concerns and Information please contact our EU
representative GPSR@taylorandfrancis.com
Taylor & Francis Verlag GmbH, Kaufingerstraße 24, 80331 München, Germany

www.ingramcontent.com/pod-product-compliance
Lightning Source LLC
Chambersburg PA
CBHW070712220326
41598CB00024BA/3119